Max Nicolai Appenroth, María do Mar Castro Varela (eds.)
Trans Health
International Perspectives on Care for Trans Communities

[transcript]

We thank the Simmons & Simmons LLP for funding this important project and the Aktionsbündnis gegen Homophobie e.V. for their support in the process of publishing this book.

Thank you to Freya Medley and Vivian Schotte for copy-editing and Karen Bennett for translating the Spanish chapters to English.

We also thank transcript Independent Academic Publishing for the cooperation and special thanks to the organization Knowledge Unlatched for the opportunity to publish this book open-access.

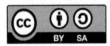

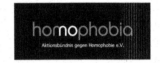

Bibliographic information published by the Deutsche Nationalbibliothek
The Deutsche Nationalbibliothek lists this publication in the Deutsche Nationalbibliografie; detailed bibliographic data are available in the Internet at http://dnb.d-nb.de

First published in 2022 by transcript Verlag, Bielefeld
© Max Nicolai Appenroth, María do Mar Castro Varela (eds.)

Cover layout: Maria Arndt, Bielefeld
Proofread by Freya Medley
Translated by Karen Bennett (Spanish Chapters to English)
Printed by Majuskel Medienproduktion GmbH, Wetzlar
Print-ISBN 978-3-8376-5082-2
PDF-ISBN 978-3-8394-5082-6
https://doi.org/10.14361/9783839450826
ISSN of series: 2625-0128
eISSN of series: 2703-0482

Printed on permanent acid-free text paper.

Contents

Glossary

Cis (or cisgender) is the term used to describe people whose gender is congruent with the sex assigned to them at birth. Cis people can be critical of and question stereotypical gender images, but subjectively they do not feel any dissonance between their gender identity and the sex assigned to them at birth.

Cis-Normativity is the assumption that everyone identifies with the sex assigned to them at birth and that there are only two sexes – female and male. Due to cis-normativity, people whose gender is different from the sex assigned to them at birth encounter a variety of individual and structural barriers and discrimination in the course of their lives. The **gender identity** of cis people is usually not questioned, as long as their gender performance is in line with the norm. Trans and gender diverse people, on the other hand, continuously find themselves in situations where they have to justify their identity and fight for its recognition.

Deadname is the first name given to a trans or gender diverse person (usually by their parents at birth) before their transition. Many trans and gender diverse people reject this name for themselves and decide to use a new name. Questions about the previous name are often considered inappropriate or invasive by trans and gender diverse persons.

Gender is the socially constructed idea what it means to be a 'woman' or a 'man'. This description includes not only one's own **gender identity**, but also the gender roles that are perceived and reproduced in our society through language, external characteristics and behavior. The lived and performed gender does not have to match the sex assigned at birth.

(Physical) Gender Affirmation describes the process that some trans and gender diverse people go through in order to align their body to their lived gender. This may include, for example, undergoing hormonal treatment (→**gender affirming hormone therapy**), hair removal and/or surgery on the primary and/or secondary sexual characteristics, or speech therapy for the voice, among other options. It is important to note that this process is individually designed and that there is no predetermined sequence of steps that an individual 'must' undertake. Each person decides individually to include or exclude certain steps. Linguistically, the concept of affirmation expresses what is meant: the affirmation of the lived gender. This process has historically been called a 'sex-change'. This term is considered unhelpful because it does not describe the actual process and it is not inclusive of the diversity of gender identities and how they are physically manifest. The term 'gender reassignment' is rejected by many trans and gender diverse people for the reasons mentioned above. Usually, the term affirmation refers to physical characteristics, but it can also describe a social or legal affirmation process →**transition.**

Gender Identity comprises those aspects of personal identity that relate to an individual's lived and experienced gender. In cis people, gender identity is congruent with the sex attributed to the person at birth. In trans and gender diverse people, gender identity deviates from this and can include identification with a different gender. This does not (always) have to happen in one of the common, binary patterns described by terms like 'female' and 'male', as well as 'female-to-male' or 'male-to-female'. People may also have gender identities between or outside binary gender norms (for example as **non-binary** or **gender fluid**). Contrary to the stereotypical assumption that gender identity is stable and unchangeable, it can change multiple times over the life course of a person.

Gender Fluid describes a form of identity that is not based on clearly defined female or male characteristics but moves between or beyond these boundaries. An identification of a person between or outside binary gender norms can be fluid and change from time to time or from situation to situation and is not a permanent state. See also **non-binary**.

Genderqueer similar to gender fluid persons, genderqueer describes a gender identity outside gender binary norms. See also **non-binary**.

Gender non-conforming similar to gender fluid, genderqueer or non-binary persons, gender non-conforming describes a gender identity outside gender binary norms and/or reject normative gender attributes.

FtM The acronym stands for 'female to male' and is often used to describe people who were assigned female gender at birth but are male.

Heteronormativity describes the assumption (accepted by the majority in the Global North) that there are only two sexes (female and male) and that appropriate romantic and sexual behavior occurs only between females and males. The consequence of this basic assumption is that people who live a sexuality outside of this norm must actively express this in order to receive (in the best case) recognition. A continuous representation of heterosexual couples and families in the media and language consolidates this basic assumption.

Gender Affirming Hormone Therapy (GAHT) is the process of taking drugs containing testosterone or estrogen (often in combination with testosterone blockers) in order to align a trans or gender diverse person's body with their gender identity. Not every trans and gender diverse person decides to undergo this step of a physical transition. Also known as Hormone Replacement Therapy (HRT).

Hysterectomy is the surgical removal of the cervix.

Indigenous Gender Diverse Identities In many global regions gender diversity is present, accepted, if not even celebrated since hundreds, if not even thousands of years. Through the Christian colonization of the world those identities have been oppressed, marginalized, and often almost eradicated. Some identities are: Transpinays/Transpinoys/Baklâ (Philippines), Brotherboys/Sistergirls (Australia), Fa'afafine (Samoa), Hijras (India), Kathoey (Thailand), Māhū (Hawaii/Tahiti), Muxes (Mexico), Two-Spirits (North America), Vakasalewalewa (Fiji), and many more.

International Classification of Diseases (ICD) is a diagnostic manual published by the World Health Organization (WHO) that is used and recognized in WHO member states. The ICD-10, the currently dominant version of the manual, still categorizes trans identity as 'transsexualism' and lists 'gender identity disorder in children' as a mental disorder. In the updated version of the ICD-11 gender diversity has been moved to a new section of sexual health related matters and it was renamed to 'gender incongruence of adolescence and adulthood' and 'gender incongruence of childhood'. The update to ICD-11 in happened in 2019, however, this most recent version of the classification will only come into effect on January 1st, 2022.

Intersex describes people who were born with physical and sexual characteristics that do not fit the stereotypical norm of male and female. These can be variations in the body's hormone composition, primary and/or secondary sexual characteristics, internal sexual organs and/or chromosomes that differ from the normative patterns of a 'female' and 'male' body. Intersex people sometimes are also trans.

Legal Gender Recognition (LGR) is the process of changing one's name and/or gender marker on official documents (i.e., ID card, passport, driver's license and where possible, also on birth-certificates). LGR is not available in many countries/regions and in some countries trans and gender diverse people are still legally persecuted.

LGBTQIA+ stands for Lesbian, Gay, Bisexual, Trans, Queer, Intersex, Asexual and more (+). The acronym often appears in connection with trans-relevant topics and describes in the broadest sense the community of people with diverse experiences of sexuality and gender.

Mastectomy is the surgical removal of the breast tissue. In many cases this also includes a reshaping and replacement of the nipples. This procedure is colloquially called top surgery.

MtF stands for 'male to female' and is often used to describe people who were assigned male gender at birth but are female.

Non-Binary (also enby) describes a gender identity outside the binary gender norm of female and male. Some non-binary people may have a stronger tendency towards a female or male identity, but do not see themselves 'completely' as either a woman or a man. Non-binary people are often mistakenly categorized together as if their genders are the same. However, there are an infinite number of non-binary gender identities and they do not fall on a spectrum 'between' female and male; rather, each gender is unique to the person.

Many non-binary people regularly experience being misgendered since, due to cis-normativity, other people constantly assume that they are either female or male and cannot even imagine that they might be neither.

Passing is when a trans and gender diverse person's lived and performed gender is correctly read and understood in their environment. Trans and gender diverse people who are 'passing' are perceived by most people around them to 'fit' with the gender they are. The term 'passing' is considered problematic by some trans and gender diverse people because it reinforces the idea that trans and gender diverse people can have their gender identities respected only if they reshape their appearances to conform absolutely to cis-normative ideas of what a 'man' or 'woman' should look like.

Phalloplasty is the surgical procedure of shaping a penis. This procedure is colloquially called bottom surgery.

Ovariectomy is the surgical removal of the ovaries.

Queer as a term originates from English and means: strange, suspicious, crazy. Originally the term was used as a derogatory term for LGBTIQA+ people. However, in the 1980s, LGBTIQA+ activists began to use the term provocatively and affirmatively for self-representation. This redefined 'queer' as a positive self-description from within the community and this step led to a gradual wider acceptance. 'Queer' studies, for example, is today a well-established academic discipline. The term queer is used more and more as an affirmative term describing, among others, people who live outside heterosexual and/or cis norms, or who question normative structures of sexual and gender identity.

Sexual Identity Contrary to gender identity, which describes a congruence or even an incongruence with the lived/performed and ascribed gender, sexual identity (also called sexuality) refers to the desire of a person. It describes to whom we feel emotionally, sexually and/or romantically attracted. Like gender identity, a person's sexual identity can change over the course of a person's biography. Moreover, contrary to societal assumptions that a lived physical sexuality always aligns with emotional preferences and/or sexual fantasies, these can in fact differ. In addition to homo, bi- and heterosexuality, which are conceptually situated within the gender binary, there are pansexuality, omnisexuality or an identification as 'queer' or 'bi+'. These latter terms are considered more inclusive since they describe desire in a way that can include people of all genders, not just people of the 'same' or the 'opposite' gender to oneself. People may self-describe as asexual if they do not live a (physical) sexuality. Contrary to stereotype, asexual people can and do have close romantic and intimate partner relationships. The sexual orientation of a trans person can change during/through a transition, but primarily sexual orientation has no relationship to the gender identity of an individual.

TERF stands for Trans-Exclusionary Radical Feminist and describes people who actively oppose trans and gender diverse rights and specifically promote the exclusion of transfeminine identities. One of their claims is that trans women are not women and therefore should be excluded from women's spaces. Most feminists reject this notion and are critically opposed to TERFs. TERFs have united with conservative and right-wing groups to further push an anti-trans-agenda, especially in the UK.

Trans and gender diverse is used in this book to describe people whose gender is different from the sex assigned to them at birth. The word trans with an open ending is a term chosen by the community itself and covers a variety of identities. Trans and gender diverse people may seek physical affirmation and/or legal recognition of their identity (where this is an option). There are trans and gender diverse people who find themselves in the binary framework of female or male; but many trans and gender diverse individuals also have gender identities outside these categories (→ **non-binary, genderqueer, genderfluid**). Some people who are living as a different gender compared to the sex assigned to them at birth speak of their trans identity as something that happened in the past and are not (or no longer) trans or gender diverse. They often describe themselves as women or men with trans and gender diverse experience or a trans and gender diverse history.

Transphobia describes discrimination and violence towards trans and gender diverse people. However, the term transphobia mischaracterizes this behavior as an individual aversion or phobia, when in fact it is a socially-sanction pattern of violence towards trans and gender diverse people that is reproduced at individual, familial, social, economic, legal, and institutional levels. Rejection and/or violence towards gender diverse people requires active participation and a conscious decision to exclude or attack. By contrast, phobias are (mostly) uncontrollable states of fear and a phenomenon on which those affected are usually unable to exert any active influence. Some more accurate alternative terms are trans and gender diverse antagonism or trans and gender diverse hostility.

Transition describes the process of a trans and gender diverse person adapting to their lived gender on a social, physical and/or legal level. This affirmation takes place individually for each person and can involve one or more steps. Some trans and gender diverse people decide for themselves only one type of social transition (e.g., change of first name, pronouns, external appearance – i.e., in the form of different clothing) without desiring a legal or medical transition. Others may wish to transition on various levels. It is important to note that it is only the individual person who determines what the desired steps are. There is no 'right' or 'wrong' way of a transition. Additionally, in many countries, laws exist that hinder trans and gender diverse people's ability to transition, and in some countries, trans and gender diverse people are legally and socially persecuted if they attempt to do so.

Transsexuality is a term often rejected by people from the trans and gender diverse community because it was originally coined in the 1950s by cis doctors to distinguish between supposedly 'healthy' (cis) and supposedly 'sick' (trans) people. The term is therefore pathologizing since it is still associated with the diagnosis of a mental disorder. In addition, the term is criticized because the ending '-sexuality' is misleading. Being trans or gender diverse refers to the **gender identity** of a person and not to their **sexual identity**. Given the diversity of the trans community and the large number of possible identifications, some trans and gender diverse people nevertheless choose this term for themselves, as they feel it to be their own and it is often easier to convey this term.

Vaginoplasty is the surgical procedure of shaping a vagina. This procedure is colloquially called bottom surgery.

Introduction

Max Nicolai Appenroth & María do Mar Castro Varela

About This Book

The publication of an international book on trans and gender diverse health is the first of its kind and an empowering and uniting momentum for the community. By sharing cross-regional experiences, we wish to broaden the landscape of looking at trans health by not favoring a perspective dominated by the global north. Trans and gender diverse people are rarely given the opportunity to speak up for themselves, and their unique perspectives of the authors in are what make this publication so valuable. The majority of contributions are written by trans and gender diverse identified authors. It is important to give the community a voice and to let personal experience speak, where the topic is so personal and concerns the bodies of individuals. We wish to thank and express our gratitude to all contributors for having made this project possible.

The diversity of bodies and identities draw our attention toward hegemonic ways of seeing and thinking and of how we systematize and organize what we see. This is especially evident in an area such as healthcare, which remains, after all, strongly influenced by normative body images. Navigating healthcare as a trans and gender diverse person comes with a number of obstacles. Aware of these barriers, trans and gender diverse people across diverse cultural and national contexts often seek healthcare in the metropolis, hoping that the anonymity of a bigger city and the promise of progressiveness will secure them an appropriate and dignified treatment. People who differ from dominant gender norms and/or choose non-normative life practices may also seek refuge in the city, where they are less likely to be noticed and questioned about their being. Lobby groups have not only drawn attention to particular experiences of discrimination but have generally started to demand a life characterized by that is not "governed like that, by that", to put it in Michel Foucault's words (see Foucault 1997: 28). Whenever those people who are turned into minorities scandalize their marginalization and stigmatization and demand to be allowed to live differently – as long as nobody's life is hurt by it – everyone benefits. Even cis people, who say that they are satisfied and happy with the gender they were assigned at birth, are able to represent, interpret and perform gender in a more heterogenous way when the world has been made safer for trans and gender diverse people. Struggles against social injustice are always struggles for democratization. The manifold criticism that comes from trans and gender diverse movements and Trans Studies not only points to a medicine that continues to disempower those who do not conform to stereotypical gender norms. This criticism also excoriates the forced standardization of gender and sexuality coming from the field of medicine. When we talk about trans and gender diverse health and care, it seems to us that it is paramount also to talk about self-care and to document resistance to a care work that actually does not care, but humiliates or even hurts people. Trans Studies also encourage us to question the normative guidelines of gender and to demand more from a political and ethical point of view than the view that we are only worthy of care if we conform to gendered norms. It should be possible to break the standards without being rejected, ridiculed and stigmatized.

In this sense, the book is to be understood as a strategic-political book. On the one hand, the contributions problematize unquestioned social norms, state regulations, institutional ignorance and narrow-mindedness towards gender diverse people, which results in the production of suffering in many ways. On the other hand, the book addresses ways in which care work, care provision and general perspectives on trans and gender diverse people can be shaped in a community-oriented and inclusive way.

Trans and Gender Diverse Health: Not Redeemed

The human right to the "highest attainable standard of physical and mental health" is one of the economic, social and cultural Human Rights formulated by the UN in the Economic, Social & Cultural Covenant of 1966, Article 12 (Wulf 2016). It was ratified by the majority of countries world-wide. However, many people de facto suffer from insufficient healthcare. They fall ill more often and have a lower life expectancy overall. For this reason, the importance of the topic of trans and gender diverse health must be addressed whenever one seeks social justice. The situation of trans and gender diverse people vis-à-vis care institutions globally is a genuine scandal. In some countries, things are moving very slowly in the direction of justice and inclusion of people of diverse genders. Argentina, for example, has one of the world's most ample trans rights laws. The so-called "Gender Identity Law" was passed in 2012 and turned Argentina into a country where people are allowed to legally change their name and gender marker without having started gender affirming hormone therapy and without the need to present a psychiatric diagnosis. This development is of course, on one hand, due to the fact that trans and gender diverse communities world-wide have become more visible in fighting against injustice. The de-pathologizing of trans and gender diverse experience is the goal of many community advocates. In 2019 the WHO removed being trans and gender diverse from the list of mental disorders International Classification of Diseases (ICD-11), moving it into a separate chapter called "Conditions Related to Sexual Health". However, it will probably take some time for the ICD-11 first, to be translated into many different languages and then be implemented internationally. As it stands, trans and gender diverse people around the world continue to be diagnosed with a mental disorder, often as a precondition for receiving medical care or legal recognition.

Moreover, in many countries gender diversity is almost invisible within the medical and social care system. Although trans and gender diverse equality has been able to attract greater attention worldwide, the provision of care for trans and gender diverse people remains problematic and fragmentary at best – while in the worst cases, as documented in some of the contributions to this book, it is discriminatory and harmful.

Care Situation of Trans and Gender Diverse Persons: The Great Unknown

Although little is known about gender diversity in general, the topic has gathered interest in recent years, especially within the English-speaking academic literature of the global north. Nevertheless, the present volume is one of the first to provide perspectives on trans and gender diverse healthcare from diverse geographic regions. It attempts to give a comparative overview of the medical, (psycho-)therapeutic and nursing care, as well as self-care, of trans and gender diverse people. Moreover, it aims to stimulate further debate, studies, and theoretical considerations.

There is still little knowledge about how trans and gender diverse people are cared for and, above all, how good care institutions work to fulfill their duty vis-à-vis trans and gender diverse people. On top of that, there are hardly any studies about the negative experiences of trans and gender diverse people in care settings.

Barriers that trans and gender diverse people encounter in their search for healthcare services include stigmatizing (psycho-)therapeutic treatments, over-pathologization, reduced access to gender-specific medical services (gynecological/urological examinations, treatment for infertility and others), refusal of public and private health insurance providers to cover the cost of transition-related services and, at times, complete refusal of medical services. These and many other barriers make access to good (medical) care difficult for trans and gender diverse people.

Often the barriers to accessing nursing or medical care are not immediately obvious. A lack of knowledge on the part of staff about the needs of gender diverse people, as well as a lack of respect for trans and gender diverse patients – sometimes even openly displayed transphobia, lead to, to say the least, insecurity on both sides. It is not uncommon that a practitioner displays a boundary-crossing curiosity, putting the patient (sometimes unintentionally) into the role of an 'expert' without them having given their consent. In situations in which people seek help from doctors, therapists, psychosocial counsellors, caregivers or other people in the healing and nursing professions, being 'interrogated' is perceived by those affected as violent and humiliating. In short, in their search for medical treatment, trans and gender diverse people cannot rely on being treated professionally and respectfully. Trans and gender diverse people rather expect to be treated disrespectfully, being confronted with massive ignorance.

Often problems start the moment that a trans and gender diverse person seeks an appointment, since registration forms ask for gender and name. In most countries, these forms only offer two options for gender (M/F), denying trans non-binary (and intersex) identified people the right to a respectful description of their identity. When the first name of a trans and gender diverse person does not seem to match with their outward appearance or the name on their insurance card, it leads often to shameful discussions. Further inquiries are rarely conducted with appropriate sensitivity.

Trans and Gender Diverse-Inclusive Language

Social change is always also accompanied by a change in hegemonic language practices. The use of language in regard to gender diversity has changed considerably over the past 100 years. The well-known physician Magnus Hirschfeld, an outspoken advocate for sexual minorities and first advocacy for homosexual and trans rights spoke of a "third gender" already at the beginning of the 20th century. The term "transsexuality", on the other hand, was first mentioned in a scientific publication much later, in 1949, to distinguish between supposedly 'sick' people, those who describe a gender variance for themselves, and 'healthy', non-trans people. We reject the use of the term "transsexuality", as it is part of a pathologizing practice, and it also often wrongly implies the sexual preferences of a trans and gender diverse person. Being trans or gender diverse refers to gender identity and not to a person's sexual desire. Unfortunately, these two things are commonly confused leading to misconceptions about the identity of trans and gender diverse people and their sexuality.

Over the past few years, the word trans has become more and more established, not only within trans-activist contexts and within the trans and gender diverse community. For the present anthology, we have decided to use trans and gender diverse as terms that describe people whose gender is different from the sex assigned to them at birth. The ending after trans is deliberately left blank to leave room for the self-description of an individual. Trans is often used as a single term but can and is often combined with other terms. Possible variations are: transgender, trans non-binary, genderqueer, trans-fluid, gender non-conforming, etc. (see glossary in this volume). Due to the uniqueness of gender experiences, there will be always new terms and/or alternative combinations of terms.

We also want to point out that the concepts of trans and gender diversity can be understood in various ways. The terms trans and gender diverse are predominantly used in the global north. The concept of a gender binary, and even the simple idea of "trans" may not be adequate in countries with a long history of gender diversity.

Historically, trans and gender diverse people play an important role in indigenous cultures across the globe. Examples for other terms for gender diverse persons and communities are: Aranu'tiq, Kathoey, Muxe, Fa'afafine, Burrnesha, Two-Spirit, Sekhet, Brotherboys & Sistergirls, among many others.

Structural Barriers to Transition Related Care & Legal Gender Recognition

Legal gender recognition (LGR) describes the measures some trans and gender diverse people take to align their lived gender identity with the description in legal documents, such as ID cards, passports, and/or birth certificates. This may include changing one's name and/or gender marker. Not every trans and gender diverse person wishes to engage in the process of LGR, for various reasons. For example, in most countries, the legal gender options remain limited to the binary of 'female' or 'male', meaning that for non-binary and other gender diverse people, there is no option to have their gender legally recognized. Thus far, only Malta, Aotearoa/New Zealand, India, Pakistan, Argentina, the Netherlands, Denmark, Australia, Germany, Nepal, and some states in the United States allow a gender marker on legal documents other than 'female' or 'male'. In some countries, like in Germany for example, the third gender option is reserved only for intersex people who can provide a medical statement about a physical gender variation. Trans and gender diverse people who are not born with an intersex variation cannot officially benefit from the third gender option called "diverse."

Every year Transgender Europe (TGEU) collects information about the legal regulations concerning trans rights in 49 continental European countries and 5 Central Asian countries. According to the latest TGEU statement, a total of 31 states have legal gender recognition regulations in place. However, 44 countries still demand a mental health diagnosis before allowing changes to legal documents. As TGEU points out, "the diagnosis requirement contributes to stigma, exclusion, and discrimination and relies on the false notion that being trans is a psychiatric disorder" (TGEU 2021). Additionally, 8 out of the countries that have measures for LGR in place still require a (forced) sterilization from individuals who wish to align their documents. To demand permanent infertility from trans people has been found to violate Human Rights of an individual by the European Court of Human Rights.

As these examples from Europe show the bodily integrity of trans people is regulated by state policies. The requirement for a mental health diagnosis in combination with the forced sterilization of trans and gender diverse people who wish to change their name and/or gender marker on legal documents, is an unmistakable sign of the dehumanization gender diverse persons experience.

Many trans rights advocacy groups globally demand the possibility for LGR and name change procedures to be solely based on self-determination. As mentioned above, Argentina became the first country worldwide to allow trans and gender diverse people to change their legal identification documents based on self-determination in 2012. In Europe, Belgium, Denmark, Iceland, Ireland, Luxembourg, Malta, Norway, and Portugal have followed this example. While the relentless work of trans advocacy groups has brought some progress, other countries have rolled back trans inclusive legislations. In December 2020, Hungary discarded a law that allowed Hungarian trans and gender diverse people to legally transition.

Even though a physical transition is not the goal of all trans and gender diverse people, many trans and gender diverse people who are seeking a formal change of first name and gender marker also decide to engage with gender-affirming medical treatment. To obtain hormones that are not produced by the body to a sufficient degree can be difficult and time-consuming, often because of gatekeeping by medical providers. For example, in many countries, a report from a therapist is a mandatory precondition for gender affirming hormonal treatment. In consequence, some trans and gender diverse people try to avoid this by purchasing hormones from informal sources (e.g., via the internet or from unknown sources), a practice that can have serious health consequences. Hormonal treatment requires regular medical supervision, and self-treatment carries the risk of infection and incorrect dosage. Where androgen blockers and estrogens can often be administered orally in form of pills or dermally through creams, testosterone in many cases is injected intramuscularly. It is often not possible for people who wish to receive this treatment to purchase clean injection material. Knowledge about self-administration with hormones is often acquired online or based on the experience of other trans and gender diverse people in the local community. The information is not always sufficient, and bodies differ in needs, which can lead to complications.

In most countries that offer reimbursement for transition-related care covered by health insurance, further examination processes and long waiting periods (from a few months to several years) have to be faced by those who decide in favor of gender affirming treatment. Even the application process for compensation usually requires multiple certificates from physicians and therapists. Going through the several stages of 'assessment' can be experienced by trans and gender diverse people as disempowering and disrespectful of their life choices.

The Big Knowledge Gap

There is still a lack of studies on gender diversity and an absence of items on (trans-)gender identity in population-wide surveys. In consequence, it is not possible to provide exact data about how many people are trans or gender diverse. Current studies from the U.S. suggest that about 1.4 million U.S. Americans (0.6% of the total population) are trans or gender diverse (Flores et al. 2016). A study in the Belgian region of Flanders found among 4,304 respondents that 2.1% of respondents had an ambivalent feeling about their gender identity and 0.7% had a different identity compared to the gender they were assigned at birth (van Caenegem et al. 2015). Furthermore, there are many communities in the global south which have known non-binary identities for centuries without them being recognized by the different nation-states and sometimes are rather unknown in the West.

A further problem in estimating how many people are trans or gender diverse is also due to the fact that sometimes a trans and gender diverse identity is not lived openly or is not recognized as such. Many trans and gender diverse people are open with their identity and live their everyday life without hiding it. However, this does not apply to all gender diverse people. Due to concerns about or experiences of exclusion, discrimination and violence, many trans people still hide their identity. Where this identity is lived openly, it often remains dependent on situation and context. Some trans and gender diverse people live openly as trans and gender diverse among their friends or in the family but hide their gender identity at school or at work, in order to avoid discrimination. As national and international studies have shown, trans and gender diverse people are affected by discrimination and violence in school, vocational training and at work. Although trans people in Europe and the USA have an above-average level of education, this is rarely reflected in their income levels – trans and gender diverse people are found to a much greater extent in lower income groups and many live in poverty (James et al. 2016; FRA 2020).

Trans Health During a Global Pandemic

Covid-19 brought various challenges to the majority of people worldwide. Trans and gender diverse people, along with other minorities, are believed to suffer disproportionally during this pandemic. Access to healthcare (incl.

transition related care) for gender diverse individuals often necessitate traveling to bigger cities. Due to lockdown measures in many countries, travel has been restricted and, additionally, many people may avoid crowded places (e.g., trains, buses, healthcare facilities) out of fear of a Covid-19 infection. Moreover, often transition-related care is not considered as essential care and is therefore cut off (Fedorko, Ogrm & Kurmanov 2021). "Surgeries that had taken years to secure were often being delayed or cancelled, as were pre- and post-surgical care" (ibid.). A recent global study among 4,412 trans people showed that 40.5% were concerned about how the pandemic will affect their access to gender affirming hormone therapy. Additionally, this study showed that 44.2% were already living with a chronic condition (i.e., HIV, COPD, Asthma, cardiovascular diseases, back problems, among others). Out of fear of discrimination, 22.2% would not go to get tested for Covid-19, even if they displayed symptoms (Trans Care Hamburg 2020). The impact of gender-affirming care on trans and gender diverse individuals is often very much underrated, and the distress arising from inaccessibility of such treatment has severe ramifications for the affected individual. At this stage we cannot foresee the consequences resulting from many months of lockdowns, compromised access to healthcare, delayed preventive screenings, and the mental health impacts of social distancing and self-isolation. However, early indications are that existing barriers to care faced by trans and gender diverse people have been exacerbated by the Covid-19 pandemic.

This Book

For some trans people things are getting better: laws in many countries changed in favor of trans and gender diverse people, but in most of the countries worldwide the discrimination in the field of care is still very rampant. There are still lots of studies needed as we need more direct activism raising awareness of the different needs of trans and gender diverse people. This volume is a modest contribution. We hope it will lead to more awareness and future studies on the topic.

References

European Union Agency for Fundamental Rights (FRA; 2020): LGBTI II – Survey Data Explorer. [online]. Available at: https://fra.europa.eu/en/data-and-maps/2020/lgbti-survey-data-explorer (Accessed: 7 October 2021).

Fedorko, B.; Ogrm, A. and Kurmanov S. (2021): Impact assessment-COVID-19 and trans people in Europe and Central Asia [online]. Available at: https://tgeu.org/wp-content/uploads/2021/01/impact-assessment-covid19-and-trans-people-in-europe-and-central-asia.pdf (Accessed: 9 February 2021).

Foucault, M. (1997): "What is Critique?", in: The Politics of Truth, eds. Sylvère Lotringer and Lysa Hochroth, New York: Semiotext(e): 23-82.

James, S.; Herman, J.; Rankin, S.; Keisling, M.; Mottet, L. and Anafi, M. (2016): The Report of the 2015 U.S. Transgender Survey[online]. Available at: http://www.transequality.org/sites/default/files/docs/usts/USTS%20Full%20Report%20%20FINAL%201.6.17.pdf (Accessed: 7 October 2021).

Trans Care Hamburg (2020): Results [online]. Available at: https://transcarecovid-19.com/results/ (Accessed: 7 October 2021).

Transgender Europe (TGEU; 2021): Trans Rights Europe & Central Asia Index 2021 [online]. Available at: https://tgeu.org/wp-content/uploads/2021/05/tgeu-trans-rights-map-2021-index-en.pdf (Accessed: 8 April 2022).

van Caenegem, E.; Wierckx, K.; Elaut, E.; Buysse, A.; Dewaele, A.; Van Nieuwerburgh, F.; De Cuypere, G. und T'Sjoen, G. (2015): Prevalence of Gender Nonconformity in Flanders, Belgium. In: Archives of Sexual Behavior 44(5), pp. 1281-1287.

Wulf, Andreas (2016): Das Menschenrecht auf Gesundheit" [online]. Available at: http://www.bpb.de/internationales/weltweit/menschenrechte/231964/gesundheit?p=all (Accessed: 7 October 2021).

"The law is not going to tell us how to care for the patient." – Health Professionals and the Argentine *Gender Identity Act*

Anahí Farji Neer

Introduction[1]

In May 2012, the Argentinian Congress approved Law 26.743 on Gender Identity. This legislation allows any person of legal age to change their name and gender on their identity documents by carrying out a personalized procedure before the civil registry offices, without requiring judicial, medical or administrative authorization. Article 11 of the law, entitled "Right to free personal development", stipulates that any person of legal age who so wishes may access free medical treatments to "adapt their body, including their genitalia, to their self-perceived gender identity," with the sole requirement being a signature confirming informed consent. Based on the concept of comprehensive health, the legislation incorporates these benefits into a Compulsory Medical Plan, which covers Argentina's three health subsystems (public, private and social services). Before its approval in this legislation, genital surgery to align the body with gender identity could only be performed with judicial authorization, under the provisions of Law 17.132 on the Exercise of Medicine. Similarly, per Law 18.248, persons requesting the correction of registration of name and sex on their identification documents needed judicial authorization. This authorization required an extensive range of medical and psychological professionals to indicate that the person suffered from "Transsexualism" or "Gender Identity Disorder".

---

1   This article was translated from Spanish to English. A preliminary version of this paper is Farji Neer, Anahí (2018): Los/as profesionales de la salud frente a la Ley de Identidad de Género argentina. Tensiones entre el saber experto y el cuidado integral. In: Physis: Revista de Saúde Colectiva, 28(3), pp. 1-18.

The content of the Gender Identity Act was developed entirely by trans organizations in Argentina, who demanded the elimination of diagnostic and judicial requirements previously in force to access these rights.

This paper deals with the reception of the *Gender Identity Law* by health professionals in the Metropolitan Area of Buenos Aires, Argentina. It investigates the criteria that were adopted by health professionals after the approval of the Law to evaluate the admission and results of surgical interventions and hormonal treatments requested by the trans population. Between 2014 and 2019, during my doctoral and later my postdoctoral research, I conducted a total of fifteen interviews with health professionals working in the Buenos Aires Metropolitan Area with experience in gender affirming treatments requested by the trans population. They included professionals from the specialties of mental health, endocrinology, plastic surgery, urological surgery, gynecology, phono audiology and medical clinics. In the interviews, participants were asked about their professional careers, how the Law on Gender Identity had changed the organization of care, and their perceptions of the depathologizing paradigm embodied in the Law. Each interview lasted approximately forty-five minutes and was conducted after the signing of an informed consent form. Interviews were recorded, loaded into software for the analysis of qualitative data and encoded based on the analysis dimensions indicated. In this paper, I analyze the interviews of four professionals of the specialty of endocrinology, two of mental health, two of urological surgery and two of plastic surgery.

Below, I explain the start and development of the diagnoses of Transsexualism and Gender Identity Disorder, and their incorporation into widely circulated and dominant diagnostic manuals in the local and global medical community. Then, I describe three shifts identified in the discourses of the Argentine medical field following the approval of the Law on Gender Identity: from diagnosis to counseling, from protocol to personalization-customization, and from minimization of risk to cost-benefit calculation. In the conclusions, I summarize the research and reiterate the main findings.

From the Doctor's Office to the Street: The Birth and Transformation of a Diagnosis

The birth of transsexuality as a medical and identity category associated with various medicalized interventions can be understood as a result of the advancement of endocrine knowledge and improvement of surgical techniques (see Hausman 1995). The term "psychic transsexualism" was coined in 1923 by the German physician Magnus Hirschfeld, who developed the two-tier-theory (*Zwischenstufentheorie*). The term was taken up in 1949 by the American physician David Cauldwell, who described it as an inherited organic predisposition that, combined with a dysfunctional upbringing, could produce a variety of psychological effects among which would be the belief of belonging to the "other sex". He understood it as a condition that could improve or even be cured through psychological treatment (Cauldwell 2006).

In the late 1960s, Harry Benjamin, a German endocrinologist based in the United States, established the basis for diagnosing what he called true transsexualism. In contrast to previous approaches, from his perspective, surgical and hormonal interventions could constitute an indicated therapy for such diagnostic pictures. These developments were embodied in a series of protocols applied in the mid-1960s in the Gender Identity Clinics created in the United States and later replicated in various parts of the world.

In 1979, Benjamin edited the Standards of Care for Gender Identity Disorders (SOC), in which he established a standardized method for the diagnosis and treatment of transsexualism. Initially, the diagnostic process involved ruling out psychosis and schizophrenia, then identifying three criteria: the feeling of belonging to the opposite sex, the early and persistent use of clothing of the opposite sex without an erotic sense, and contempt for homosexual sexual behavior. After the diagnostic process, treatment consisted of three progressive and inseparable stages: psychological, hormonal, and finally, surgical. In the 1980s, first Transsexualism and then Gender Identity Disorder were included in the world's most widely circulated classification manuals of mental illnesses and disorders: The Diagnostic and Statistical Manual of Mental Disorders (DSM) of the American Psychiatric Association and the International Classification of Diseases (ICD) of the World Health Organization.[2] After Benjamin died in 1986, the SOCs – which, like the aforemen-

---

2   The first version of the International Classification of Diseases dates back to 1893. In its 6th version of 1948, it included a chapter on mental disorders and in its 8th version of 1965 it included a section on Sexual Deviations, incorporating the categories of Transvestism and Homosexuality. ICD 9 of 1978 eliminated the Homosexuality category but included the diagnosis of Transsexualism within the Sexual Deviations section. In 1992, ICD 10 was published. There, Transsexualism, along with non-fetishistic transvestism and gender identity disorder in Childhood, were placed within the umbrella category of gender identity disorder (GID) (located in the chapter on Mental

tioned diagnostic manuals, are periodically revised – came under review by the World Professional Association for Transgender Health (WPATH). In its 7th edition, published in 2011, the SOC introduced concepts that recognized multiple identities and bodily possibilities, in a way of depathologizing trans identities that reflected longstanding demands from trans activists around the world (Coll-Planas 2010; Suess Schwend 2010). This document states that gender variability (or gender nonconformity) and gender dysphoria are not necessarily linked phenomena. With the terms gender nonconformity or gender variability, the document refers to those forms of gender identification or expression that differ from established cultural norms. Gender dysphoria is the term used to refer to "discomfort or distress that is caused by a discrepancy between a person's gender identity and that person's sex assigned at birth (and the associated gender role and/or primary and secondary sex characteristics)" (WPATH 2012:2). In line with these transformations, the DSM-5 (published in 2013) devoted a specific chapter to Gender Dysphoria, which is split from sexual dysfunctions and paraphilias. The Gender Dysphoria chapter mentions gender nonconformity, specifying that it does not necessarily involve an experience of psychic suffering.

Until 2012 in Argentina, requests for a change in official records and identification documents, as well as access to gender affirmation surgeries, required juridical authorization as established in the Penal Code, Law 17.132 on the Exercise of Medicine and Law 18.248 which regulates the right to the name one is allowed to use. Until the end of 2010, these legal proceedings required a psychiatric diagnosis of Gender Identity Disorder (Cabral 2003; 2007; Farji Neer 2013; 2016). Argentina's trans organizations, formed in the mid-1990s, denounced these procedures as violating the human rights of trans people. Additionally, reports prepared by these organizations demonstrated that before the *Gender Identity Law* came into effect, trans people often avoided health consultations due to experiences of mockery and mistreatment by professionals and administrative staff (Berkins and Fernandez 2005 Berkins 2007; Frieder and Romero 2014). This was addition to the bureaucratic barriers

---

and Behavioral Disorders). The 1980 DSM III also eliminated the category Homosexuality and created a new category: Sexual Identity Disorder. It incorporated the diagnosis of Transsexualism. In the 1994 version, it replaced it with gender identity disorder, which, together with Paraphilias and Sexual Dysfunctions, formed the Sexual and Gender Identity Disorders section (Di Sengi 2013).

caused by a lack of access to documentation accurately reflecteing the gender identity of a patient. These barriers discouraged and hindered access to healthcare, leading to widespread use of risky practices such as the injection of silicone oil, clandestine cosmetic surgeries and the consumption of hormones without medical supervision (Berkins and Fernandez 2005; Berkins 2007; Frieder and Romero 2014).

The *Gender Identity Act* created social and legal conditions that permitted expert discourses of medicine to be challenged by the demands of trans people. As a result, on an organized and individual scale, trans people have demanded greater participation in decision-making regarding their treatments and intervened in the instituted forms of medical authority and doctor/patient relationship.

In order to address changes and continuities in medical criteria after the introduction of the *Gender Identity Law*, I describe the approaches of health professionals who performed or evaluated the admission to hormonal and surgical gender affirmation treatments in the Buenos Aires Metropolitan Area. I analyze how the criteria for admission, the indication for treatment and the evaluation of the results were defined after the approval of the Law. At the same time, based on the interviews conducted, I identify a set of discursive changes with respect to the criteria of care present in the diagnostic manuals and international healthcare guidelines for the trans population in force prior to the 2010s.

From Diagnosis to Accompaniment

Between 2014 and 2019, most of the professionals interviewed provided interdisciplinary care in public and private clinics as well as in social security clinics. Some of the teams preexisted the *Gender Identity Law* and others were formed after its enactment, either on the initiative of individual professionals within these teams, or that of institutional medical directors. The teams were coordinated centrally by a professional who belonged to the specialty of psychiatry, urological surgery, plastic surgery or endocrinology. This was the person in charge of organizing work across these different specialties. In some instances, the teams conducted admission interviews, evaluation and referral of patients. It is worth noting that neither the Law nor its regulations, nor the National Ministry of Health through ordinances or other regulatory instruments, established a care model. Each team developed their own care guides based on local and international guidelines, accumulated clinical experience and the conceptions and criteria of their members.

One of the main guidelines for structuring care was the comprehensive evaluation (physical and psychological) of patients, to determine the extent to which they were prepared to initiate the requested treatments, especially surgical ones. The criteria that were previously intended to certify the diagnosis of Transsexualism or Gender Identity Disorder were put to the service of a more holistic process of assessment. Professionals considered that a comprehensive evaluation was necessary to understand the physical, emotional, and psychological conditions of potential patients.

The evaluation of patients had several objectives. The principal objective was to understand or help build the applicant's understanding of their identity and, from there, offer the various options available for body reconstruction, reporting the potential benefits and risks. Interviews were aimed at determining whether the person was *emotionally fit* to undergo the treatments. As the psychiatrist coordinating one of the teams stated:

> "What we do is assess the need of each person and based on their particular need, we assist them. But first we clarify their present life circumstances, that the person is clear who they are and what they need and based on that, we provide whatever type of treatments – hormonal, surgical, total, partial – it's different in every particular case" (John, psychiatrist).

In order to make these assessments, the team constructed contextually elaborated indicators of stability or instability in decision-making throughout life. An endocrinologist described the method developed as follows:

> "Talking to him and asking him for his story first, his family support, his social support, his involvement with paid work, his level of acceptance within his environment, seeing what he looks like, whether he looks like a man or a woman, how he dresses and asking him about his expectations, if he has had any other treatment in the past and trying to assess... certain patterns can tell you about the person. For example, a people who says to you 'I started law school and I quit, I started architecture and I quit, I started medical school and quit, I like the theatre but I haven't done it consistently, then you can infer that they will not be constant in their treatment" (Miguel, endocrinologist).

The evaluation was based on professional perceptions of the life trajectory of those seeking treatment. After the first interview, psychotherapeutic consultation could be mandatory or optional, depending on the criteria used by the team or the professional. In some teams, psychotherapeutic consultation was mandatory as some type of surgical intervention were required. If the person was already in therapy, the practitioners did not request that they see a different therapist, but rather requested to contact their current therapist and carry out a joint evaluation.

Despite the demands of local and international activism for the depathologization of trans identities (see Coll-Planas 2010; Suess Schwend 2010), between 2014 and 2019 in various services of the Metropolitan Area of Buenos Aires the requirement to have an endorsement by a mental health professional remained mandatory for access to genital surgery. Health practitioners maintained the need for such an endorsement by appealing to the irreversibility of interventions, speaking in a tone that seems halfway between care and guardianship:

> "There is something that simply I won´t change: the fundamental role of psychology and psychiatry. Because some people tell me now 'I don't need [psychological assessment], according to the Law.' And I say 'How do we go back from a surgery like this one? Impossible. So, we have to make sure you're okay with the surgery. If we make you a woman, how do we go back? Impossible [...] If you've already been in treatment somewhere else two or three years back, well, [we ask] for a certificate from the other psychologist or psychiatrist to say that you are fit to operate" (Raul, plastic surgeon).

If hormone treatments were requested, the indication of psychotherapeutic consultation depended on the health practitioner's criteria, depending on each case. Interview with a mental health professional was not intended to corroborate a diagnosis or to rule out psychosis or schizophrenia as in the first protocols developed by Benjamin but to assist the patient with their decision-making process regarding treatments. It also served to provide health practitioners with reassurance regarding the emotional stability of the applicants and their degree of certainty about requested treatments. Following the passage of the *Gender Identity Law*, the interview process was no longer about discharging the health professional's legal responsibility or complying with protocols, but rather a matter of professional moral responsibility, grounded in the notion of care and holistic medicine. A surgical urologist said:

> "As a doctor, it's not pleasant to operate on someone and instead of helping them, you complicate their life. Most of the messages we receive are like

'Doctor, thank you, you changed my life', it's not very nice to receive 'Doctor, my brother killed himself because of what you did to him'. So it's no longer a legal issue, it's a medical issue. We want to do things to improve people's lives, and it wouldn't be very nice to know that you operated on someone, that it's irreversible, and that the person regrets it" (Gerardo, surgical urologist).

Those who did not request psychotherapeutic consultation used evaluation mechanisms developed based on subjective criteria and, if they identified evidence of doubt or instability, implemented various forms of deterrence intended to delay intervention. Referring to the process pre-surgical consultation, a plastic surgeon said:

"I don't make them [go to therapy]; I don't ask them. What's more, I'm not a psychologist obviously, but in the conversation, I look at the profile of the patient, and for example, some patients come and I see them as very unstable and I don't say 'No!', but I say 'Look, it would be good to take time with such an important decision, why don't you come... let's take a few months and speak again.' So, I try to draw out the process when I see that the person is very unstable" (Alejandra, plastic surgeon).

The request for consultation with a mental health professional when patients do not consider it necessary constitutes a mentoring practice. The fact that mental health professionals, specifically psychiatrists, occupy a decision-making place in access to genital surgery through pathologizing practices and discourses has been called "gatekeeping" (see Lane 2018). In some respects, the arguments put forward by the health practitioners interviewed seem to express typical "gatekeeping" attitudes. However, they have other characteristics that differentiate them. The practitioners do not speak in terms of diagnosis but consider consultation with a mental health professional – not necessarily a psychiatrist – as a guarantee to safeguard the health of patients from irreversible surgical interventions. On the other hand, it is worth noting that the requirement for consultation with a mental health professional seems to be usually motivated by the doubts and uncertainties that the destabilization of gender binarism produces among health practitioners, rather than the actual health needs of trans patients.

The main challenge in avoiding power dynamics between practitioner and patient is to carry out a process of dialogue that constructs informed consent. It requires the implementation of modalities of care in which professionals recognize trans users as fully autonomous and not as subjects who must be cared for differently from any other patient who presents for medical consultation.

From Protocol to Personalization – Customization

Another of the displacements identified was the change from a model of protocolized care composed of three linear and successive stages (psychotherapy – concurrence – genital surgery) to a model of personalization or customization of treatments according to the needs of trans patients. For the medical professionals interviewed, this modality maximized the likelihood of "successful" interventions, not only in organic-functional but also in symbolic terms. Symbolic, here, refers to bodily self-representation and sexual pleasure. As explained by one of the surgical urologists interviewed:

> "It's not just surgery. Surgeons are used to thinking about surgery and nothing else, but if you start to say that this is to remove the testicles, remove the penis, make a vagina... It has a lot of symbolism. We need to talk to the patients first. Not all patients want the same type of surgery. There is a strong theme of customization and individualization here" (Mariano, surgical urologist).

Professionals assumed that to be successful they needed to develop a sensitivity that exceeded mere technical capabilities: it required attentive and committed listening to the needs and expectations of trans people. There was no protocol that could supplement the sensitivity necessary to carry out the task, since it implicated identity and sexuality, practices that were essential for the subjective constitution of each person. In this regard, when referring to mastectomies, a surgeon who was interviewed referred to the following:

> "Every patient is different, and every patient has been an apprenticeship. That learning is not easy because there are unique conditions that set the direction with each patient: the characteristics of the skin, if they are using hormone therapy, if they have used a binder or sash anything before, are all questions... the size of the breast... the patient's desire, because the patient sometimes wants a particular technique and you have to adapt it to the extent that you can [...] there are patients who come and tell me 'I don't want anything, I don't want any memory of my previous life, I don't want an areola,

I don't want a nipple, I do not want anything.' Other patients, due to the size of the breast you have to do a particular technique and then you have to do a reconstruction to create an areola and a nipple [...] It's a combination of so many factors. You have to negotiate all the time and come to an agreement" (Alejandra, plastic surgeon).

From Risk Minimization to Cost-Benefit Calculation

In WPATH protocols in force until 2011, the main risk to be weighed was that of regret, which in extreme cases could lead to suicide (Pragier 2011). But between 2014 and 2019 care was provided taking into account a wide range of possible risks, not just the risk of repentance. A multiplicity of possible consequences was weighed, including the consequences of non-intervention. Professionals began to scoff at the idea that there could be an ideal situation where there was no risk. From this perspective, they considered that both intervention and non-intervention had some kind of cost or risk to consider, whether physical or subjective. This is explained by an interviewee:

"There is a lot of commotion among medical professionals saying 'if you are going to give someone estrogen you are predisposing them to thrombosis, if you are going to give them progesterone you are predisposing them to breast cancer and osteoporosis [...]. So, they're usually thinking of the ideal, that is, of *their* ideal... 'Better if I don't give them anything and I exempt them from risk.' But they forget that if you leave someone in their present condition you have another risk. Therefore, realistically you have to take risks because if you have a person who is not happy with their sex, you have to choose between the risk of deterioration of their mental health and the risk of thrombosis, there is no option of no risk" (Miguel, endocrinologist).

In the same vein, another professional stated:

"Among people on whom I have operated, no one has expressed regret... among cases I have seen presented at conferences, there is a small percentage of people who express some small regrets [...]. I believe that with time and with the times we are living in, we're going to encounter regret sometimes. I think so. It's logical, because insofar as they go, they come, they do, they undo... well, it's going to happen. It's what I think, it's a thought of mine" (Alejandra, plastic surgeon).

For this professional, regret was an inescapable consequence given the complex experiences of trans people, who were conceived as people in constant search, fluctuation and experimentation with body and identity. For the professional interviewed, regret should be seen as one possible consequence within the multiple possibilities created by the availability of gender-affirming medical treatments for trans people.

Important questions emerge from the discursive shifts identified above. One is, who weighs up the risks of treatment options and who has the final say about which course of action to follow? The Gender Identity Act legalized gender affirming medical treatments for trans people and thus eliminated the potential for treating professionals to be accused of violating the Medical Exercise Act (*Ley de Ejercicio de la Medicina*). Nonetheless, based on the idea that there is no ideal situation and that there are always risks to consider, many medical professionals continued to exercise authority over the definition of the course of treatments, appealing to their responsibility for ethical-professional care and irreplaceable clinical experience and knowledge.

In this sense, the professionals interviewed were critical of the content of the *Law on Gender Identity* and of any legislation that aimed to intervene in the exercise of their profession. They criticized a formulation of the concept of patient autonomy that understood the patient as an individual consumer of biotech goods and services, where clinical criteria were deemed unnecessary:

> "The law will not tell us how to care for the patient, nor say when is the appropriate time to give what assessment, nor when it is time to give approval to operate, nor when treatment is not appropriate. Everything you have, everything your doctor does, has indications, counter-indications, side effects, etc. [...] There are a lot of issues that contraindicate, and while there is the Law, there are medical questions too [...] people believe that if it says in the law that doctors have to give X and Y, then suddenly the doctor is a kiosk operator who is planted there and the patient comes and says: 'Give me this, give me that' [...] well then it's like you as a doctor *do not exist* and you do not have any role" (Luis, endocrinologist).

Promises for the future: the Return to Biology

In a manner that traverses the three discursive shifts identified above, some of the medical professionals interviewed displayed a persistent interest in the scientific revelation of the supposed biological underpinnings of the existence of trans people. According to some of the professionals interviewed, although they had not yet been revealed by genetic research, a set of organic determinants – presumably genetic – would eventually be found to explain trans experiences. This is how one endocrinologist put it:

> "There must be something that makes a three-year-old boy say, 'I feel like a girl'. There's gotta be something discovered to explain that, within in fifty years, I reckon. Everything has to have a reason. Like, of premature ejaculation it's known that, some studies say that, it has a genetic basis: there are genes that have to do with the speed of the ejaculation reflex, as well as serotonin levels. Everything is regulated by genes, so something must have generated this issue. Afterwards, there's what it has to do with society" (Luis, endocrinologist).

In the same vein, another interviewed endocrinologist stated:

> "I think there is a strong biological determinant in this trans [...] it's a subject that interests me a lot: the determinant. Because understanding it would help to clarify this issue for the general population. It's not a whim. Whoever wants to be trans does not choose it, this I want to say [...] I believe that the literature in general accepts and has some evidence for the biological, for the biological determinants" (Julian, endocrinologist).

According to the interviewees, scientific confirmation of the existence of biological determinants of trans experience would provide the necessary arguments against those who understand the gender affirming treatment needs of the trans population as a "whim". At the same time, such an explanation would allow progress in social acceptance and fulfillment of the rights of trans people, since socially the argument of biological roots would bear more weight than those made in terms of inclusion and human rights.

These arguments about the scientific basis of medical practice were articulated with a feeling of hope linked to the belief that we may know, in a not-too-distant future, the organic causes that would explain the multiplicity of trans experiences. Faith in the scientific narrative operated among some health professionals as a guarantee of certainty that minimized the uncertainty and moral conflict presented to them when responding to requests for access gender affirming care. In this sense, for the professionals interviewed, the promise of the future of a still nonexistent scientific truth prevailed above the voices of the real subjects about their present vital needs.

Final Reflections

This paper discussed the reception of the *Gender Identity Law* by health professionals in the Metropolitan Area of Buenos Aires who specialized in gender affirming hormone and surgical treatments. Several discursive mutations were identified in the criteria for the entry and evaluation of the results of these treatments compared to those previously in force. These discursive mutations reflect a process of local reappropriation of diagnostic manuals and care guidelines in global circulation.

The first section addressed the birth and development of diagnoses of Transsexualism and Gender Identity Disorder, and their incorporation and transformation into the main widely circulated diagnostic manuals in the local and global medical communities. This section also set out the criteria for admission and care in force in the medical protocols that since the end of 1970 systematized standards and criteria for gender affirming medical treatment.

The subsequent three sections analyzed the main discursive mutations identified among the health professionals interviewed: from diagnosis to accompaniment, from protocol to personalization-customization, and from risk minimization to cost-benefit calculation. These mutations developed within the framework of the Argentine *Gender Identity Law*, which dejudicialized and de-pathologized access to gender affirming treatments. However, other explanatory factors were also identified, including changes in diagnostic manuals in global circulation, advancement in the acquisition of rights by LGBT people, and increasing visibility of the demands of trans groups in local public space.

In a manner that traverses the three discursive shifts identified, there was a persistent interest from the professionals interviewed in the scientific unveiling of the alleged organic basis for the existence of trans people. The expectation that these scientific certainties will be found in the not-too-distant future minimized uncertainty and moral conflict among health professionals when responding to requests for access to gender affirming-care by trans people.

Based on the analysis carried out, it can be said that the demands made of the medical community by local and global trans activists have, in some cases, managed to destabilize the certainties of health professionals and prompted a review of their practices. In other cases, medical professionals have responded with the reaffirmation of their authority in a defensive sense. Two dimensions are worth noting in this regard. On the one hand, professionals demand to be recognized as experts in their professions, and not as mere "vendors" of hormones and surgeries. On the other hand, the request for consultation with mental health professionals is the manner they have found to deal with the doubts and uncertainties that the destabilization of gender binarism causes them. This requirement to have authorization by a mental health professional to be able to access gender affirming care reproduces a 'gatekeeping' logic that restricts the autonomy of trans patients, the very autonomy that the Law on Gender Identity was intended to promote.

Taking into account these tensions, it can be said that in order to promote non-gatekeeping practices in health services, medical professionals must reflect deeply on the fears and uncertainties that gender affirming treatments provoke in them. They must implement dialogic processes of building informed consent, in which by suspending their authority, they recognize trans people as fully autonomous and not as subjects who should be subjected to differential care.

References

American Psychiatric Association (2013): Diagnostic and Statistical Manual of Mental Disorders (5th ed.). Washington, DC: American Psychiatric Association.

Barbosa, B.C. (2015): Imaginando trans: saberes e ativismos em torno das regulações das transformações corporais do sexo. Unpublished PhD Thesis. São Paulo: Universidade de São Paulo, Faculdade de Filosofia, Letras e Ciências Humanas.

Bento, B. (2006): A reinvenção do corpo: sexualidade e gênero na experiência transexual. Rio de Janeiro: Garamond.

Berkins, L. (2007): Cumbia, copeteo y lágrimas. Informe nacional sobre la situación de las travestis, transexuales y transgéneros. Buenos Aires: ALITT.

Berkins, L. and Fernández, J. (2005): La gesta del nombre propio: Informe sobre la situación de la comunidad travesti en la Argentina. Buenos Aires: Ed. Madres de Plaza de Mayo.

Cabral, M. (2003): Ciudadanía (trans) sexual. Artículo sobre Tesis premiada. Proyecto sexualidades, salud y derechos humanos en América Latina [online]. Available at: https://programaddssrr.files.wordpress.com/2013/05/ciudadanc3ada-trans-sexual.pdf (Accessed: 11 November 2021).

Cabral, M. (2007): Post scriptum. In: Berkins, L.: Cumbia, copeteo y lágrimas. Informe nacional sobre la situación de las travestis, transexuales y transgéneros. Buenos Aires: ALITT, pp. 140-146.

Cauldwell, D. (2006): Psychopathia Transexualis. In: Stryker, S. and Whittle, S. (Eds.): The transgender studies reader. New York: Routledge, pp. 40-44.

Coll-Planas, G. (2010): La policía del género. In: Missé, M. and Coll-Planas, G. (Eds.): El género desordenado. Críticas en torno a la patologización de la transexualidad. Barcelona: Egales, pp. 55-67.

Dean, M. (1998): Risk, Calculable and Incalculable. In: Soziale Welt, 49, pp. 25-42.

Di Segni, S. (2013): Sexualidades. Tensiones entre la psiquiatría y los colectivos militantes. Buenos Aires: Fondo de Cultura Económica.

Farji Neer, A. (2013): Fronteras discursivas: travestismo, transexualidad y transgeneridad en los discursos del Estado argentino, desde los Edictos Policiales hasta la Ley de Identidad de Género. Unpublished Master Thesis. Buenos Aires: Universidad de Buenos Aires, Facultad de Ciencias Sociales.

Farji Neer, A. (2016): Sentidos en disputa sobre los cuerpos trans: los discursos médicos, judiciales, activistas y parlamentarios en Argentina (1966-2015). Unpublished PhD Thesis. Buenos Aires: Universidad de Buenos Aires, Facultad de Ciencias Sociales.

Farji Neer, A. (2018): Los/as profesionales de la salud frente a la Ley de Identidad de Género argentina. Tensiones entre el saber experto y el cuidado integral. In: Physis: Revista de Saúde Colectiva, 28(3), pp. 1-18.

Foucault, M. (1999): ¿Crisis de la medicina o crisis de la antimedicina? In: Estrategias de poder. Barcelona: Paidós, pp. 343-361.

Frieder, K. and Romero, M. (2014): Ley de identidad de género y acceso al cuidado de la salud de las personas trans en Argentina. Buenos Aires: Fundación Huésped y Asociación de Travestis, transexuales y transgéneros de Argentina.

Hausman, B. (1995): Changing Sex: Transsexualism, Technology, and the Idea of Gender. Durham: Duke University Press.

Lane, R. (2018): "We Are Here to Help". Who Opens the Gate for Surgeries?. In: TSQ: Transgender Studies Quarterly, 5(2), pp. 207-227.

Pragier, U. M. (2011): Trastorno de identidad de género (TIG), un enfoque integral. In: Revista de la Sociedad Argentina de Endocrinología Ginecológica y Reproductiva, 18(2), pp. 45-56.

Suess Schwend, A. (2010): Análisis del panorama discursivo alrededor de la despatologización trans: procesos de transformación de los marcos interpretativos en diferentes campos sociales. In: Missé, M. and Coll-Planas, G. (Eds.): El género desordenado. Críticas en torno a la patologización de la transexualidad. Barcelona: Egales, pp. 29-54.

World Professional Association for Transgender Health (WPATH, 2012): Standards of Care (SOC) for the Health of Transsexual, Transgender, and Gender-Nonconforming People (7th ed.) [online]. Available at: https://www.wpath.org/media/cms/Documents/SOC%20v7/SOC%20 V7_English2012.pdf?_t=1613669341 (Accessed: 11 November 2021).

The Context of Health for Guatemalan Trans People[1]

Alex Castillo & Yusimil Carrazana Hernández

Universal access to health is understood as "the possibility for all people to have access to the health services they need, with due quality and regardless of their socioeconomic status, ethnicity, place of residence, sexual preference, religion or culture" (ACCESA 2015:9). Universal access to health also includes the idea that in order to access health there should be no payment or payments that jeopardize the financial stability of people or households.

Universal health stems from the principle that health is a human right and applies not only to providing health services but in ensuring the conditions that allow people to be healthy.

"In such a way, universal access to health involves an approach in which the health system, and not just the system of provision of services, must be seen in its complex relationship with other systems (educational and economic, among others) to become the object of analysis and transformation." (ACCESA 2015:7)

Therefore, ensuring the human right to health of all people refers to the idea of taking affirmative commitments and actions on behalf of people who are the most vulnerable, due to various factors such as gender and ethnic discrimination. For trans people, reflections on the social determinants of health have illustrated that gender-based violence impacts access to healthcare. We also know that discrimination in the education and economic system creates vulnerability for trans people because it conditions them into violent contexts or contexts in which they cannot access healthy lifestyles.

Health services in Guatemala have not yet managed to be efficient, supplied, have full coverage, good care and generate positive outcomes for the

---

1   Original text was submitted in Spanish and translated to English.

most vulnerable people to access them. This is due to deep and historical problems ranging from racism and structural sexism—by concentrating all services in the mestiza/ladina capital—to corruption and low tax revenue, which makes quality and supplied services impossible.

According to the Alliance for Universal and Public Access to Health (ACCESA) (2015) there are three historical roots for understanding the state of the health system in Guatemala: The political root constitutes the political decisions that mark the type of state that is Guatemala, highlights a state of counterinsurgency state before the Peace Accords—a process that ended 36 years of internal armed conflict—where, in the context of the Cold War, it was not appropriate to expand and improve public services. After the Peace Accords the state was decreased, with the result being an increase in the privatization and precarity of state workers. This resulted in services being inefficient and institutions not responding to the population, and instead co-opted by political interests.

When we talk about racism and structural sexism, we refer to the political, economic and social factors that undermine the right to healthcare of those populations affected by racism and sexism. As mentioned above, political factors refer to public decisions that have weakened public institutions or made the state work against people—such as in a counterinsurgency state. It is no coincidence that in Guatemala, women and indigenous peoples, among other groups that have been oppressed (i.e., trans people), do not find functional public institutions to access health services.

The economic root to understanding the state of the health system in Guatemala is that dominant social groups are not interested to invest in human capital for their workforce. This is because the economic models of elites do not depend on skilled labor, which in turn depends on a healthy and educated population. Additionally, a monoculture business, the extractive industry, etc. do not motivate governments and elites to advance the health system because these economic activities do not require educated, healthy and technically qualified populations (ACCESA, 2015).

Finally, there is a social root to health problems. It is found in the history of Guatemala, as its colonial origins created the conditions for inequality in Guatemalan society, based on the diverse ethnicities and skin color of its inhabitants. This history generates an ideology that legitimizes and justifies social inequalities in access to health. This ideology is not only ethnocentric, it is also heterosexist and patriarchal because it prioritizes the bodies it esteems as white, heterosexual, cis and knowledgeable. The three main roots above complement each other, as a social context of discrimination legitimizes both political violence and unjust economic decisions based on identity. In turn, political decisions have been aimed at sustaining this economic system rather than generating a welfare state.

This context is very similar to the rest of the Central American region, few variants are issues of access to healthcare of trans people. Central America shares a similar geopolitical history determined by social inequality, institutional weakness, and an ultraconservative colonial elite.

The Differentiated and Comprehensive Health Strategy for Trans People

In response to the above-described fatal health situation the *Differentiated and Integral Health Strategy for Trans People* 2016-2030 arose. The strategy seeks to generate affirmative actions for trans people to have access to public health. This strategy is focused and generated by trans civil society organizations and seeks to avoid the segmentation of health services because the trans population suffers from stigma, discrimination and poor attention in the health system. Since no country in Central America allows legal gender recognition, there is no legal framework that protects this population in the region.

The guiding principles of the strategy are in accordance with the principles of the Yogyakarta Principles and are also justified on the basis of the principle of universal and free health for all people as a human right. It has the following priority areas:

Area I. Disease Prevention and Health Promotion
Area II. Comprehensive Care
Area III. Institutional Strengthening
Area IV. Monitoring and Evaluation, each with its general and specific objectives.

The strategy arose from a recommendation from international agencies to the state of Guatemala in 2013. Subsequently, trans organizations began working on the content of the strategy and in 2015 it was signed indicating a political will by the State of Guatemala. It should be noted that in 2015 the Government was in transition in an election year and the minister of health back then cut off a large part of the strategy's content and passed on its implementation to the next government.

The operation of the strategy has been inefficient and the public health system in Guatemala has not prioritized a reform to the administration of the health system since the administration does not currently tie health sub-systems under clear objectives or generate transparent, functional administrations. The country's widespread political instability has also caused little clarity in Guatemala's health policy, as in 2017 the health minister at that time resigned because of a political crisis of corruption of the current government.

The country's macro policy has direct impacts on the non-implementation of the strategy, as institutions such as the Ministry of Public Health and Social Assistance (MSPAS) do not operate correctly . Corruption translated into opacity in public spending, clientelism to appoint people in technical posts and co-opted trade unions that prevent internal meritocracy within the ministry's employees are some of the reasons for the malfunctioning system.

To date, the differentiated and comprehensive health strategy for trans people has not been operationalized efficiently. Despite some advances such as the distribution of responsibilities within MSPAS and the progress of a communication strategy for development (ECD). This latest strategy, however, has been carried out with abuses and trans people have stated that, despite existing evidence of insufficient knowledge on trans health within the ministry, the MSPAS refused to take responsibility for educating its staff and interpreted the content of the ECD as healthy lifestyles for trans people.

To operate the strategy, an institutional strengthening process must be carried out and political clarity must be made in the need for universal access to health as a human right. Facing this institutional gap, the transmasculine community in Guatemala self-organized to respond to their basic health needs.

In addition to this problem, we encountered health professionals who have not had any academic training regarding the needs of the trans population, since it does not exist in any medical student curriculum. Medical providers continue to stigmatize trans people as 'abnormal' and interpreting their existence as 'a sin'. They mostly refuse to pay attention to this population's need based on their religious beliefs and ignorance.

The Health of Trans Men in Guatemala

In 2019 the Trans-Training Collective of Trans Men conducted an exploratory study among trans men (Martínez & López 2019) mostly urban middle-class 'mestizos'. Regarding access to healthcare, 32% reported to consult private doctors when getting sick, 24% seek medical help in private hospitals, 28% go to public hospitals, while the remaining 20% do not receive medical care of any kind (Martínez & López 2019:26).

These data respond to the general deficiencies of the public health system in Guatemala. However, the study shows that of 31 reports of trans men, who experienced discrimination in health facilities. Another 65% of this population said they faced discrimination also in public services (Martínez & López 2019:26). These results show how the health system subdivides the population not only by social class and the ability to pay for medical bills, but by gender identity.

The Trans-Training Collective, in addition to following up on the health strategy for trans people, has also started to offer comprehensive and specific drop-in days, to meet urgent needs among the transmasculine population.

Among the data collected in 41 medical records(Martínez & López 2019), the following most common problems for transmasculine health needs could be identified: 1) Self-administration of gender-affirming androgen hormones (i.e. testosterone) for masculinization with consequences on the health of the circulatory system; 2) Urinary tract infections, often asymptomatic, as a side effect of testosterone use in the body; 3) Triglycerides and high cholesterol, often as a result of poor diet, but also in correlation to gender-affirming use and; 4) Polycystic ovaries as a side effect of increased testosterone in the endocrine system (Martínez & López 2019:26).

Added to physical symptoms, mental health problems have to be addressed. More than half of the fifty participants expressed feelings of some form of anxiety, sleeping issues or suicidality. Only 32% considered mental health as something important in their lives. This has been negatively affected as two suicide attempts have been reported (as of June 2019) within the transmasculine population which were not mentioned in the study.

Lastly, it is important to note that the transmasculine community does not trust medical institutions. Based on experiences of discrimination in healthcare settings, trans men prefer to receive healthcare services by the Trans-Training Collective meanwhile seeking medical help in the public healthcare system is considered to be the last option. These concrete micro approaches demonstrate that if we focus on the general access to health services in Guatemala there is a clear institutional debt to the Guatemalan population visible.

Comprehensive Healthcare of the Trans-Training Collective

In light of this crisis in accessing healthcare for the trans population, in 2017 the first and to date only healthcare clinic in Central America specifically for trans men and non-binary people, assigned female at birth (AFAB) was opened.

The transfemale population was not included, as the founders of the clinic the Trans-Formation Men's Collective consisted only of transmasculine and AFAB non-binary persons. However, four trans women did receive treatment, but the resources available are very scarce, which limits the functionality of this clinic.

The clinic operates only one day per month and relies on donations, as the services provided to the community are completely free of charge. The services offered are: general medicine and gender-affirming hormone therapy; individual psychological care; and focus groups, for the members of the collective and their families. Participants of these focus groups learn more about trans and gender diversity and how to face a sexist, misogynist, conservative, and religious society.

Most people served in this clinic are between 17 to 72 years (mostly between 20-30 years); lower middle-class; with average schooling; the vast majority is unemployed; and 90% reside in Guatemala City and its surroundings.

Although many identify as trans, not all have the necessary economical resources to be able to afford a physical transition. The costs of laboratory blood analysis are high and due to low or no income many can't afford gender-affirming hormone therapy with testosterone.

Focus Groups of Trans Men and AFAB Non-Binary People

Given the little or no information that the population has on the subject of trans and gender diversity and how to start a transition with caution, responsibly and accompanied by peers, who have already started the transition process, the focal groups offer a space for conversations. These conversations are accompanied by exercises that allow getting to know the personal stories of each participant opening possibilities to new members to raise their concerns and questions about the transition. The participants with experience answer in a responsible way and above all knowledgeable about the specific Guatemalan context the trans population lives in and with.

It has also been a space, where through sharing one's personal experiences empathy by other group members was felt leading to meaningful conversations and recognizing ways to deal with trauma. Many have been exposed to violence because of being trans and this space allows them to gain confidence to share traumatic experiences for the first time in their lives. This has created very strong ties of solidarity and companionship.

This self-support group serves as a form of group therapy that helps the group members to see that they are not alone, that there are more people who had the same or similar experiences in their lives and the most important thing is to learn and support each other through those experiences.

It generally takes effort, to educate on human rights, social injustices and masculinities that are not toxic. Living in a very sexist society often comes with the assumption that masculinity must follow a pattern of a traditional male role. This is difficult for our social movement because we fight to eradicate any type of violence especially based on gender.

Most of the violence trans persons in Latin America suffer comes from their families. Trying to foresee and prevent this menace, we have started a sensitization process with consenting relatives.

Similar to the group of trans men, family members come together to participate in conversations providing support, and most importantly, help to recognize their family member as a trans person. Trans family members are not seen anymore as 'abnormal' family members who have to be converted, punished, or corrected. We wish to reach the contrary, that the family becomes supportive of their trans family member, which contributes to the mental health of all involved.

The aim is to prevent further violence experienced inside the family, and also to the excusing of this form of violence. As a consequence of a normalization of violence, trans persons often experience domestic violence as 'normal', producing a feeling of guilt, and the assumption that they themselves are to be blamed for this violence – a violence they are exposed to from a very early age on.

This was demonstrated in a study (Martínez & López 2019:34) which showed that 62% of the violence experienced by trans people comes from within their own family.

Psychological Care Individually

The lack of knowledge in healthcare professionals vis-à-vis trans populations, makes it very difficult to find, for example, psychologists who support trans people. Oftentimes we need to educate them around trans issues and provide them with the few existing scientific resources about this topic.

In addition, it is well known that the processes of professional psychological support should be on a continuous basis with a regular frequency, rather than only e. g. once a month.

Based on his own personal experiences, Gabriel Alvarez, a trans man and psychologist, has promoted sexual diversity with special emphasis on the trans population in the Faculty of Psychology at the University of San Carlos de Guatemala.

Through the peer-support of a trans-identified psychologist, by now 22 trans men have been supported. Using the Burns' depression and anxiety scale instrument out of these 22 trans men, 15 have been diagnosed with anxiety, 6 with depression and 1 case with a bipolar disorder.

The 15 cases of anxiety were classified as severe and were accompanied with symptoms of acute insomnia, lack of appetite, lack of desire to live, and addictions (especially alcoholism). Anxiety was mainly caused by troubles of accepting their own trans identity and not knowing how to explain the situation to their families. The individuals expressed fear of rejection, punishment, stigma, and discrimination that they were suffering from in their everyday life.

Three cases of depression were classified as mild, based on unmet needs or unmet goals in life. The other three cases included suicidal ideation of which two already tried to commit suicide more than once.

All cases were addressed with emergency supportive therapies. Following the diagnosis specific actions were taken:

- Successful diagnosis and treatment resulted in monthly therapy and specific coordinated support in potential crisis situations.

- Cases that needed further follow-up were referred to affordable professional's support and support by the trans men collective to make sure the person continues to attend their respective therapies.

- In cases that required psychiatric treatment, the person is made to schedule an appointment with a healthcare professional and take, if needed, medication. This situation may be subject to the economic situation of the affected person. Although this type of treatment is usually covered by the state and free of charge, it was already explained in the introduction how weak and malfunctional the health system in Guatemala is in general. The affected person may also encounter healthcare professionals, who pathologize them for being trans. Cisgenderism may put them even at greater risk for harm and mental health related problems.

It is urgent that we achieve partnerships with psychiatrists who are able to support trans people and to raise awareness for the situation of this community. Unfortunately, these partnerships have not been achieved so far which puts the lives of trans people at great risk.

Medical Care

Similar, to the field of psychology, medical doctors are often unaware and reject trans people. The trans community is denied healthcare, both privately and publicly, which is a clear violation of human rights.

The State of Guatemala does not recognize the rights of the trans population, so it is common practice for the trans population not to seek medical healthcare services and to self-medicate, which puts their lives at constant risk.

In the face of this great need for attention, Dr. Yusimil Carrazana Hernández was contacted, who has to date attended to the needs of more than 80 trans men from the Central American region. Since 2017 she began to support the clinic, where trans women, trans men, and AFAB non-binary people receive general healthcare, as well as gender-affirming hormonal treatment. Although, the clinic is open only once a month, it aims to support the trans community 365 days a year.

In addition to healthcare services, Dr. Yusimil Carrazana Hernández has initiated an education program around different health issues, to raise awareness of the risks that can occur if individuals do not undergo preventive healthcare check-ups.

Gender-Affirming Care

Gender-affirming hormone therapy (GAHT) is mostly desired by the local trans community. Those who visit the monthly clinic come for this purpose. Some are prior to GAHT, and some have already started without any medical supervision, which means they suffer greater health risks.

The first requirement to start the process of GAHT in a controlled way in the clinic is the initial conversation with the coordinator of the collective. The coordinator is responsible for explaining all the consequences and potential arising difficulties dealing with family, social, religious, and educational matters in the Guatemalan context. These conversations aim to support and guide them in various different aspects affected by a transition.

The doctors evaluate the person's medical constitution and run different tests prior to a gender-affirming hormone treatment. If the test results are within normal parameters and if pre-existing conditions allow, the person is asked to fill out an "Informed Consent" form.

Once all requirements are fulfilled, the doctor indicates the dose of testosterone that each individual requires. In Guatemala, only intramuscular injectable solutions are available. Monthly monitoring is carried out and the laboratory tests are repeated quarterly. Based on these regular check-ups the continuation of treatment with hormones can be upheld.

The biggest issues faced by the community is the high cost and shortages of testosterone. At times, those issues result in that many are not able to continue their GAHT periodically or that in many cases the treatment is permanently suspended. As part of the monitoring and follow up care, ultrasound check-ups of the abdomen and breasts are performed every six months and free of charge.

Hysterectomies (the removal of the cervix) are common procedures, but not covered for the transmasculine population in public or private healthcare services. Providers often don't even know that some trans men request this type of surgery. In light of the situation, the collective has started to locate safe and friendly places for this treatment. Staff in those places are sensitized and well informed, so that the gender identity of the patients is respected by everyone involved.

Mastectomy (removal of the breast) for trans men is not covered by the state or by any health insurance, making it an almost unattainable dream for this population in Guatemala. Currently only one plastic surgeon from Guatemala performs this procedure at a cost of about $2.800. Considering that the majority of the trans population, whether professionally trained or not, lack employment opportunities. This limits their income and the little money they earn is needed for their daily life. For that reason, many transmasculine persons wear binders (often bandages to compress the breast). This method often comes with side effects. The compressions are often used for more than 8 hours daily and because they are not anatomical, nor allow the necessary ventilation for the skin they lead to skin lesions, bruising, blistering, and infections of the skin that, when not adequately cared for, could lead to serious complications. Additionally, compressions in the stomach area can cause gastric reflux or chronic gastritis. Transmasculine people are also not familiar with the culture of breast self-examination, which would help detect any anomalies timely.

Using a packer (a replica/prosthesis of a penis and testicles to create a 'bulge'; mostly made from silicone) often turns out to be an issue, too. Generally, there is little access to this type of accessories, due to high costs. Those, who had the chance to acquire a packer start using it without proper information about the required hygiene standards. Packers are often used daily for more than 8 hours and not cared for appropriately regarding hygiene. There have been frequent and repeated urinary tract infections, which were caused by the misuse of this type of prosthesis.

Phalloplasty (surgical construction of a penis) is a widely unknown subject to healthcare professionals and inaccessible in Guatemala. The only plastic surgeon, who performs mastectomies in Guatemala, stated that based on his religious principles "I would never perform this type of surgery".

Sexually Transmitted Infections and HIV

The transmasculine community in Guatemala is not familiar with existing methods of STI/HIV prevention. The risk for contracting an infection through sexual contact is though high. Taking into account that from the aforementioned sample of 50 trans men, 22% identified as bisexual/pansexual and 10% as homosexual (Martínez and López 2019:15), additional to high rates of experienced sexual violence, expose this population to STI and HIV risk. Sexual violence is often considered as a "corrective" process to avoid gender diversity.

To many populations at risk, HIV testing is for free, but not for individuals with a vagina and those who do not engage in sex work. This makes STI/ HIV testing often too expensive for the transmasculine community. In consequence, they are not performed regularly.

Educational Talks

Because of living in a conservative and highly religious society, educational talks on sexual and reproductive health are a forbidden topic for children and youth. For adults it is considered a taboo topic, because of the heteronormative and cisnormative environment. For the trans population it is an unknown and unexplored topic. Because of that the Trans-Formation Collective has initiated a series of informative talks, which help to share the knowledge about prevention of diseases related to the sexual and reproductive health.

The topics of these talks include, for example, sexually transmitted infections; Visual Inspection with Acetic Acid (VIA) and pap tests, the correct use of accessories in trans male population, and the prevention of addictions (drugs and alcoholism), etc.

Future Challenges

Being the only care clinic for the transmasculine population in Central America and working practically only on a volunteer basis, we know about the great challenges ahead of achieving sustainability of our services, since we are no longer counting on the current key players, who gave much of their time, we are likely to disappear, leaving our population at risk and without care.

It is urgent to continue working and lobbying for our community within a failed state, which does not see the trans population as a subject to human rights. But they exist and share the same obligations as the rest of its population: Health is a human right, a right that for the trans populations of Central America has historically been denied, so it has become a privilege to which few have access.

Bibliography

Martínez, S. and López, T. (2019): Estudio Exploratorio de Hombre Trans 2019 [online]. Available at: http://cceguatemala.org/wp-content/uploads /2017/06/Estudio-Exploratorio-de-Hombres-Trans.pdf (Accessed: 25 January 2022).

Access to Trans Healthcare in Russia

Yana Kirey-Sitnikova

Historical Background

The first experiments in transition-related healthcare in the Soviet Union started in the late 1960s—early 1970s. The pioneer researcher of transsexualism[1] Dr. Aron Belkin was working in Moscow with intersex, and later also transsexual, patients at that time. Some of these patients expressed a need for body modifications as an aspect of transition. Schemes of hormonal treatment were developed in Moscow by Dr. Irina Golubeva, who also performed feminizing surgeries. In 1970-1972, a series of phalloplasty surgeries was performed on a trans patient by Dr. Victor Kalnberz in Riga, Latvia, which was part of the USSR at that time. All of the doctors involved in treatment of transsexuals at this stage had extensive experience working with intersex people and used similar techniques. Dr. Belkin, although sympathetic to the needs of intersex patients, showed contempt towards transsexuals, who in his opinion, lacked the "biological basis" for their condition (Belkin 2000). Nevertheless, medical care was provided, which involved psychiatric evaluation for several years and hospitalization to a psychiatric institution.

These pioneer specialists often faced misunderstanding and even pressure from their colleagues and authorities. For example, Dr. Kalnberz was almost diagnosed as insane by a special commission sent by the Minister of Healthcare. In the end Dr. Kalnberz was reprimanded. Kalnberz was cautioned his operations constituted 'mutilation' and went against the state ideology (Kalnberz 2013). In addition to providing medical support, doctors often had to help their patients with legal gender recognition. While no official procedure existed, the process usually required sanction from the Minister of

---

1   The terms transsexualism and transsexual are used throughout this chapter, reflecting the historical context that is under discussion.

Healthcare and Minister of Internal Affairs (Kon 2008). Medical care for trans patients was mainly performed in Moscow, but since the beginning of the 1980s, when psychiatrist Dr. Alexander Buxanovskij took interest in transsexualism, Rostov-on-Don in Southern Russia became another center for trans people. A psychiatric commission for trans people was established in 1984 in St. Petersburg in the Mechnikov North-Western State Medical University.

Despite the difficulties involved, provision of medical care to transsexual patients continued. Already in 1976, the Rules for Amending the Acts of Civil Status mentioned "hermaphroditism" as a legitimate reason to change one's legal name.[2] In practice, this clause was used by trans people as well. According to Dr. Buxanovskij, "full sex conversion" included three steps in the following order: (a) changing legal sex (in accordance with the 1976 rules); (b) hormonal treatment; (c) surgical "sex-transformation" (after at least one year of hormone replacement therapy), including amputation of penis, cliteroplasty, labioplasty, sigmoid colon vaginoplasty for trans women, or mastectomy, two- or three-step phalloplasty, and hysterectomy for trans men (Buxanovskij 1994: 34f.). That means that no body modifications were required for legal gender recognition (LGR) at that time.

However, this rather progressive picture is problematized when one considers who wrote the histories of this time. In most cases, we have to cite the doctors themselves, and it is not surprising that they might try to present their practices as more humanistic than they really were. Even given this bias, doctors writings from the period describe trans people who were obliged to wait for several years to get their diagnosis and stay in a psychiatric facility for months with patients of the sex that they were assigned at birth. Sometimes these trans-friendly (for that time) doctors mention attitudes of their conservative colleagues, who diagnosed trans people with sluggish schizophrenia or performed reparative therapies. As already mentioned, medical care was available only in a few cities, which attracted patients from all over the Union. On a positive note, care for trans patients was free of charge, like all health services during the Soviet period.

Accounts of trans people which would help to reconstruct their perspective on healthcare in this period are unfortunately very scarce. The most promising source of information would be letters trans people wrote to their doctors.

---

2   "Introduction of amendments, additions and corrections to the Acts of Civil Status is performed: ... t) when surname, name and patronymic need to be amended in relation to the change of sex (in hermaphrodites)".

Some of them were published by Dr. Belkin (2000), but the majority has not been studied yet. During the Perestroika period, it became possible to talk more openly about gender and sexuality. One such example is a 1990 interview in the popular journal Sobesednik. The story begins in 1961 when a trans woman first approached doctors for medical care. The doctors mocked her and said she suffered from paranoid schizophrenia. Later she met Dr. Irina Golubeva who prescribed feminizing hormone replacement therapy (HRT). Shortly after she started gender affirming treatment, the doctor died in an accident. Other doctors refused to help her, which lead to multiple suicide attempts. In the psychiatric facility, where she was put afterwards, she experienced mistreatment and torture perpetrated by other patients. Doctors forcibly injected her with testosterone. A short time before the interview was conducted in 1990, she was finally diagnosed as transsexual and received permission to undergo a surgery. It is difficult to generalize from such scattered accounts, but the picture that seems to emerge is that transsexuals were able to get appropriate care if they approached the right doctor, while they were misdiagnosed and mistreated by the rest of the medical community (Mulina 1990).

The collapse of the Soviet Union resulted in a transition from the Semashko system[3] of centralized free universal healthcare to a mixed public-private model. To address the shortage of funds and increase competition among health providers, budgetary financing of healthcare was supplemented by Mandatory Health Insurance (MHI). Private practice and clinics were allowed (Popovich et al. 2011). As will be seen later, decentralization and privatization of healthcare provision had a tremendous impact on access to trans-related healthcare in post-Soviet Russia.

Clinical Recommendations and Guidelines

In August 1991, just a few months before the dissolution of the Soviet Union, the Ministry of Health adopted Methodological Recommendations on the Change of Sex, coauthored by Dr. Belkin (Belkin and Karpov 1991). The recommendations were based on Harry Benjamin International Gender Dysphoria Association's (HBIGDA) Standards of Care and the authors' personal

---

3   Centralized state-run and state-funded system which provided free access to healthcare to all citizens.

experience. According to the text, the doctor had two basic pathways to treat transsexualism: (1) sex reassignment (the term in Russian is *polovaya pereorientaciya*, which will be further explained later), including LGR and surgery, or just LGR, or (2) sex reconciliation, aimed at acceptance of one's sex. After the diagnosis had been issued, a one-year probation period was required before surgery. At the beginning of this period, LGR was performed, and HRT prescribed. Short-term hormonal treatment was indicated in certain cases of 'transvestism', too. On the other hand, the text recommended against performing sex reassignment to individuals suffering from alcoholism, drug addiction, those pursuing 'antisocial lifestyles' and prisoners, until they "turn to a morally and physically healthy lifestyle". These recommendations have had lasting effects on medical practices and LGR not only in Russia, but also in other post-Soviet countries.

On 6 August 1999, the Russian Ministry of Health adopted Decree N311 which introduced the Clinical Guideline "Models of diagnostics and treatment of mental and behavioral disorders". The Guideline provides general description, procedures of diagnostics and treatment of disorders listed in Chapter V (Mental and behavioral disorders) of the International Classification of Diseases-10 (ICD-10), which had been implemented in Russia on 1 January 1999. The definition of 'transsexualism' (F64.0) in this guideline excludes intersex people, while the symptoms listed include so-called 'homosexual orientation', which in this case means sexual or romantic attraction to people of the gender that one was assigned at birth. Differential diagnosis is made with schizophrenia, transvestism, homosexuality, and organic damage to the brain. Further contraindications include alcoholism, drug addiction and antisocial behavior (same as in 1991 Recommendations). The treatment is subdivided into three stages: (1) preparatory (observation by a psychiatrist for at least 2 years, psychological, physical examination, diagnostics of transsexualism); (2) sex reassignment (HRT, surgeries, amending legal sex—the order of those is not mentioned); (3) rehabilitation (follow-up observations, psychotherapy). The decision to allow surgeries and LGR is made by a commission consisting of three doctors, their specialization is not mentioned (Krasnov and Gurovič 1999).

On 13 December 2012, the guideline was repealed by the Ministry of Health (Decree N1042). To this day, no replacement has been put in place. Instead, the Standard of Primary Medical Care in the Case of Sexual Identity Disorders was introduced by the Ministry one week later. The Standard lacks detail and does not reflect the actual experiences of trans people. For example, the average length of treatment is listed as 365 days. As treatment options, it mentions only psychotherapy and HRT, and only four specific drugs are listed. Surgery is not listed as an option for treatment. Thus far, there is no evidence that the Standard has had any effect on clinical practice.

The lack of clinical recommendations provides ample scope for doctors to proceed with diagnostics and treatment as they wish. This means that there are both conservative and progressive treatments possible depending on the doctor. Many trans activists claim that such a situation gives them opportunity to advocate for improved services at the local level. On the other hand, this makes the quality-of-service dependent on the place one lives in, the ability to travel to a different region and, last but not least, access to information about friendly doctors. Although trans activists have established many online resources, where trans people can find feedback on individual doctors, the digital divide persists. This means that less informed individuals with fewer resources are obliged to endure humiliating treatment at the hands of transphobic doctors.

There have been a number of attempts on behalf of trans activists to push the Ministry of Health to adopt new clinical recommendations. The latest attempt began in June 2019 after the Ministry revised the procedure for adopting clinical guidelines, stipulating that future guidelines must be written by organizations of medical professionals. The introduction of the ICD-11 by the World Health Organization (WHO) in May 2019 has changed nothing so far. To implement the ICD-11 in Russia will take several years. Providing a correct translation and a fast implementation of the ICD-11 is another goal of the Russian trans movement.

Legal Gender Recognition

The order of steps which one was expected to undertake during transition was significantly altered in post-Soviet Russia. While in Soviet times LGR was the first step, followed by HRT and surgeries, post-Soviet Registry offices started demanding HRT and at least some surgeries (the minimal requirements were usually mastectomy or orchiectomy) as a prerequisite for changing legal gender. It is difficult to determine the reason for this change. In general, varying approaches were a result of a legal vacuum. The 1991 Recommendations that permitted LGR before any medical interventions were not legally binding. Furthermore, they were issued by the Ministry of Health, while the Registries were under the Ministry of Justice. This legal vacuum was supposed to be filled by the Federal Law N143 "On the acts of civil status" (1997), which states in Article 70 that the person's records can be amended on presenting "a document of the established form about the change of sex issued by a medical organization". This law did not state whether the "change of sex" refers to one's psychological, hormonal, or morphological sex. The actual "established form" of the document, which could clarify this matter, was expected to be devised by the Ministry of Health. However, the Ministry did not clarify it for the following 19 years. As a result, registry offices in different regions of the country had varying practices of LGR, but in most cases the diagnosis 'transsexualism', HRT and some surgeries were required (Kiričenko 2011). In many regions, trans people had to sue the registry to have their gender recognized.

LGBT organizations in Russia have demanded for years that the Ministry of Health clarify what the "established form" of documentation required for LGR would be. This lack of clarity and its negative consequences were mentioned in the Ombudsman's Report in 2011. On the other hand, not all activists supported the introduction of a clear set of requirements, fearing that in the conservative political context any specific LGR procedure that was developed would not be liberal enough and would only make the situation worse. Based on their opposition to being pathologized, some individuals hoped for a legal framework that would make LGR possible without the need to receive a diagnosis of 'transsexualism'.

In 2017 the Ministry of Health finally issued a relevant draft Decree (087/y). This initiative came as a surprise, not only for trans activists, but also for doctors working in the field of trans health. The draft of this decree was controversial for several reasons (Kirey-Sitnikova 2018):

• It used the undefined term *polovaya pereorientacia* (which seems to be a translation in the wider sense of the term 'sex reassignment', a literal translation would be 'sexual reorientation'). This did not correspond to any diagnosis in either ICD-10 or the beta version of ICD-11.
• It requires that an individual undergo one and a half years of psychiatric evaluation before referrals are made to a medical commission eligible to issue the 'medical document' which states that a person has undergone 'sexual reorientation'.
• These medical commissions may only be established by a medical organization with licenses in both psychiatry and sexology. Only a few organizations in Russia have licenses in both fields.

- The 'medical document' issued by the commission would be valid for only 1 year. If a person was not able to change their legal gender during this period, they would be required apply for a new document.
- The draft contained no explicit reference to HRT or surgeries as requirements for LGR, but neither did it rule out such requirements.

Trans activists had two weeks to submit their opinion as part of the public consultation procedure. As a result of an ad hoc grassroots campaign, 73 individuals (some representing organizations) submitted comments criticizing the proposal. After a reconciliation process between the Ministry of Health and the Ministry of Justice, which was not transparent and did not include relevant stakeholders, the final version was published in early 2018. The length of psychiatric evaluation, which previously had been 1.5 years, was no longer mentioned, but the other controversial points listed above all remained. The removal of references to required length of psychiatric evaluation is sometimes described as a victory for the Russian trans movement, although the exact role played by the activists' actions remains unknown due to the lack of transparency in the process.

With the "established form of the medical document" finally in place, LGR became more or less standardized all over Russia. Trans people now have to be diagnosed with 'transsexualism' and get a medical document stating that *polovaya pereorientacia* ('sex reassignment') has occurred. No medical interventions are required. Going to court is no longer necessary. Once one applies to the registry with the medical document, it takes about a month to get their name and legal gender amended. With these details changed by the registry, it takes about 10 days to get a new passport. Unlike some other countries, in Russia trans people can change not only their passport but all other documents as well, including their birth certificate.

Diagnosing 'Transsexualism'

According to the new LGR procedure, the "medical document of the established form" is issued by a medical commission consisting of a psychiatrist, a sexologist, and a clinical psychologist. The need for a diagnosis of 'transsexualism' is not explicitly stated but it is usually assumed in practice. The diagnosis is issued by the same commission as the medical document, often at the same time. Since there are no clinical recommendations for diagnosing 'transsexualism' in place and the rules for issuing the medical document are vague, actual practices vary greatly between different medical commissions. The commissions can be classified into state-run and private. State-run commissions tend to be more conservative, while private commissions are often established by trans-friendly doctors at the initiative of activists.

Many trans people apply to be diagnosed in Moscow, where several commissions are established. The state-run Serbsky Center for Psychiatry and Narcology is a bastion of conservative attitudes to trans people, with a very strict definition of 'transsexualism'. The leading specialists are Dr. Vvedenskij and Dr. Kibrik. The City Psycho-endocrinological Center was originally established by Dr. Belkin as a state-run institution, but it is now privately run by Dr. Matevosân. Nevertheless, this Center's views on transsexualism don't differ from those dominant at the Serbsky Center. Doctors from these two organizations regularly cooperate in authoring academic articles and send trans patients from one place to another. Because doctors from these organizations are considered established authorities in treating transsexualism, many trans people visit them, if they have no information about trans-friendly options. Of the trans people who seek diagnosis through these two organizations, few succeed.

The Moscow-based Scientific Center for Personalized Psychiatry, headed by Dr. Solov'ova, was established in cooperation with trans activists. Evaluation at this Center includes initial consultations with a psychiatrist, a sexologist and a psychologist, various tests to rule out intersex conditions, as well as two meetings of a medical commission: the first one to issue a referral for surgeries and hormonal treatment; the second one to issue the 'medical document' for LGR. Both meetings can be arranged on the same day, so trans people arriving from other cities need to spend no more than 1-2 days in Moscow. The costs vary but are generally around 500 USD for diagnosis through a private commission.

In St. Petersburg there are two commissions. One of them is currently based in the private clinic of Dr. Isaev. The other is situated within the North-Western State Medical University, under Dr. Ekimov. Dr. Isaev has been working with trans patients since the 1980s. Over time his views have evolved significantly, so he is now considered one of the most trans-friendly psychiatrists in the post-Soviet region. Before 2015, Isaev's commission was situated in the state-run Pediatric Academy, but Isaev was made to resign after a campaign organized against him by anti-LGBT activists. The commission was reestablished in a private clinic, and the prices rose significantly. On the other hand, since they are no longer required to follow the Pediatric Academy's internal regulations, the commission has become more flexible and mostly issues diagnosis in less than a week. As for the commission at the Medical University, it requires 2 years of psychiatric evaluation, but it is free.

Outside Russia's two biggest cities, a number of commissions have been established in such cities as Samara, Omsk, Novosibirsk, Tyumen and Rostov-on-Don. The commission in Samara is private and was established at the initiative of trans activists. This commission is among the cheapest (approx. 250 USD) and probably the most trans-friendly commission at this time. The commission at the Center "Phoenix" in Rostov-on-Don, which is privately run, is known for its conservative attitudes. It is currently headed by Dr. Buxanovskaya, who is the daughter of Dr. Buxanovskij, one of the pioneers of trans research discussed earlier in this article.

There is a great many violations of human rights, dignity and ethical norms associated with this process of issuing the diagnosis and the medical document. These are most present in the practices of the more conservative commissions. When visiting private clinics, trans patients are made to pay for unnecessary tests and consultations. Meanwhile, in state-run institutions it is sometimes necessary to pay bribes in order to receive the correct diagnosis (rather than, for example, schizophrenia). Cases of sexual harassment and coercion are known. Some doctors require trans people to get undressed in front of the commission. There is also anecdotal evidence, for example in web forums, that trans people have been used for research purposes without their consent. Trans people are either not asked to give their informed consent for participation in research projects, or have no real possibility to say no, since they depend on the doctors to get the right diagnosis. Sometimes doctors oblige trans patients to undergo costly medical tests that are needed for the doctor's research, while having nothing to do with diagnosing 'transsexualism'. Some patients complain that the commission's decision might depend on arbitrary facts, such as physical appearance, sexual orientation or insufficient length of HRT.

Hospitalization, which used to be widespread before, is now rarely required to get the diagnosis. But there are reported cases in which doctors took bribes from relatives of trans people who wished them to be involuntary hospitalized in a psychiatric institution and undergo 'reparative treatment', which is comparable with conversion therapy. Many of these violations go unreported. They are often faced by trans individuals who are not connected to the local (or national) trans movement. If they had access to better information, it would be unlikely that they would visit these doctors. Yet since understandably, many trans people do not go public about their negative experiences, the perpetrators remain unpunished.

To sum up, in Russia a diverse landscape can be found. On one side of the spectrum, there are very liberal commissions which issue diagnosis in a couple of days and to most people who apply. On the other end of the spectrum, there are very conservative commissions with an extremely narrow definition of transsexualism, who perpetrate clear violations of trans people's rights and dignity. What is common to both settings is that trans people are required to pay to be diagnosed, whether officially in private clinics or as bribes to doctors in state-run institutions. It is generally possible to get the diagnosis and the medical document in a few days, but only if one has enough money to travel to another city and pay for the commission.

Hormonal Therapy

HRT has been provided to trans patients since the 1970s. However, due to the incompetence of doctors, some trans people received no HRT after surgeries, leading to a 'post-castration syndrome' and related health issues. These problems were often misdiagnosed. As a result, some of the trans patients had to undergo unnecessary treatment. For example, a trans woman who had her surgery in 1974 and suffered from post-castration syndrome afterwards, was erroneously diagnosed with chronic adrenal insufficiency by local doctors, who treated her with glucocorticoids, further worsening her condition. Only in 1982 did she receive the correct diagnosis and treatment in Moscow (Kozlov/Kalinčenko 1995). Dr. Kalinčenko, working in the Endocrinological Scientific Center in Moscow, has been the leading specialist in the field of HRT for trans people since the late 1990s. Treatment protocols in the Center are based on international practice. For trans women, they include estrogens (ethinylestradiol, 17-beta-estradiol or estradiol valerate) and antiandrogens (mainly cyproterone acetate, 50-100 mg/day). For trans men, standard testosterone drugs (Sustanon 250, Omnadren 250, Nebido) are used (Kalinčenko 2006).

Few endocrinologists in Russia possess sufficient competence to provide trans people with adequate care. Those doctors who have that knowledge mainly work in commercial clinics, making their help financially inaccessible for many trans people. Another issue is that the diagnosis 'transsexualism' is usually a requirement to obtain a prescription for hormone treatment. These structural and financial barriers force many trans people to take hormones without prescription or medical supervision. This practice is only possible because most pharmacies in Russia do not ask for a prescription when selling estrogens and anti-androgens (although they are obliged to do so by regulations).

The situation is more difficult for trans men, since the sale of drugs containing testosterone is strictly regulated. The prescription is valid for only one dose, meaning that trans men have to visit the doctor every few weeks and pay accordingly. It is also possible to obtain testosterone illegally. These drugs are imported from abroad and are often of poor quality, causing health complications. Further, some trans individuals have faced criminal charges for buying hormones without a prescription.

To compensate for the inadequate knowledge of the majority of doctors, many trans people immerse themselves in scientific literature and provide peer-to-peer support to others. Information is spread on the internet or provided in the form of individual consultations. Although the disseminated information might at times be outdated or incorrect, this is believed to be nonetheless more reliable than the advice provided by some ignorant doctors.

With the advancement of the trans movement in Russia the situation is slowly changing, as trans organizations work toward educating doctors. An illustrative case is the activities of the St. Petersburg-based organization T-Action. In cooperation with the Almazov Medical Research Center, they established a program of further training for endocrinologists, who wish to work with trans and intersex people. On completion of the program, the doctors receive an official certificate that is approved by the government. Besides this activity, the organization leads an ongoing project, in which trans people visit doctors as patients, talk to them about their needs and ask them to join an e-mail list for trans-friendly doctors. In spite of these efforts, the great majority of endocrinologists throughout the country remain ignorant of the needs of trans people.

Surgeries

Since the early 1990s, microsurgical techniques were developed in the Russian Research Center of Surgery (Moscow) to address the needs of trans patients. The whole range of feminizing and masculinizing surgeries is available, but their quality varies. Among 103 patients who underwent vaginoplasty in the aforementioned Research Center, 29 (28%) had complications (Kučba et al. 2014). Among 114 trans men who underwent phalloplasty in the same Center, 20 (18%) had complications (Milanov, Adamân and Kazarân 2001). A number of surgeons are working in other regions as well, although their techniques are less advanced. Some of their patients go to redo their surgeries in Moscow. Out of concern for better quality, those with more financial resources tend to choose foreign clinics, mainly in Thailand and India (trans women) or Serbia (trans men). At the same time, Moscow is a destination for some trans people from neighboring post-Soviet countries, where these surgeries are not available, or the quality is even worse.

In almost all cases, the surgeries are performed on a commercial basis. There do exist regional quotas for high-tech medical care, but there are only a few trans people who are able to benefit from them. To use this mechanism, one has to obtain a false diagnosis other than 'transsexualism', since 'transsexualism' itself is not on the list of the diagnoses eligible for this program. Orchiectomy can be obtained under Mandatory Health Insurance (MHI), but, once again, the official diagnosis should not be 'transsexualism', but 'hypogonadism' or another similar diagnosis. Before the adoption of the new LGR procedure (087/y), orchiectomy was the minimum requirement for changing one's legal gender in many regions. Since the new LGR procedure requires no surgeries, orchiectomy is performed less often.

Trans Activism and the Access to Healthcare

Trans activism in Russia, depending on definition, can be traced back to the year 2000. Expansion of the internet in Russia and post-Soviet countries made it possible for large numbers of Russian-speaking trans people to connect and build networks for the first time. Varying digital resources were established, including mailing lists, web forums and websites. These developments enabled trans people to exercise their agency as more active stakeholders in their health. Information from foreign websites (almost exclusively in English) was translated; topics included theories of the formation of gender identity, psychological matters, HRT, surgeries, voice training, cosmetics, success stories, etc. Locally important information, such as contacts of doctors, personal stories of people receiving the diagnosis, HRT and surgeries, changing their legal gender, etc., was also disseminated through these online platforms. While previous generations of trans people had to rely solely on doctors for information about medical gender-affirmation, the internet and social media became alternative sources of information, created by trans people for trans people.

During the first years, however, the mission of these resources was limited to sharing information. The next stage, starting roughly from 2009, involved the trans movement's active intervention in the sphere of trans healthcare. Several events for doctors have been organized by the initiative group FtM-Phoenix since 2009, including two large conferences in 2013 and 2014. The group was also involved in advocacy work within the Ministry of Health, in order to introduce the "document of the established form" for LGR. In 2011, a trans couple organized a clinic in Moscow that has since provided medical care for trans people, including endocrinology, surgeries and a psychiatric commission that can issue the diagnosis of 'transsexualism'.

In other cities, trans activists started direct communication with local doctors to raise their trans sensitivity. T-Action, established in St. Petersburg in 2014, organizes seminars and trainings for doctors, runs a government-approved course for endocrinologists and has written a book on trans health. Many Russian trans organizations and individual activists participated in the public discussion of the Decree leading to the new regulations for LGR in 2018. Since 2011, it has become increasingly common for activists to advocate for 'de-pathologizing' the discourse about trans experience, although the views of activists may not reflect the broader views of the Russian trans community.

Discussion and Conclusions

For a socially conservative country, which is known internationally for its human rights violations, especially against LGBT people, Russia has a surprisingly developed system of medical care for trans people. All transition-related medical procedures are available within the country, even if their quality leaves much to be desired. The procedure of LGR is among the easiest and quickest in the world and requires no medical interventions. Much of it is based on the legacy of the Soviet Union, where medical care for trans patients was being developed since the late 1960s – early 1970s and the main agents of positive change were the doctors themselves. This does not mean that the present situation goes without criticism. Since 2014, a number of bills have been proposed by conservative members of parliament (MPs) that would restrict the rights of trans people, including the right to trans-specific medical care and LGR. So far, all such proposals have failed, after being criticized by other MPs and members of the bureaucracy. The reason for the failure of these proposals is that trans issues are perceived in a medical context by most politicians and bureaucrats. The opinion of the doctors, who claim that 'transsexualism' is no different from any other illness, enjoys widespread credibility.

Viewed against the backdrop of almost 50 years of medical care for trans people in Russia, trans activism is a relatively recent phenomenon. Trans activists engage in various activities that have a bearing on trans people's access to healthcare, including education of doctors, advocacy within the Ministry of Health, as well as shifting the discourse on trans issues and promoting de-pathologization. This work has contributed to the recent liberalization of LGR, increased awareness among doctors and establishment of several trans-friendly commissions. On the other hand, some trans people fear that increased visibility of trans activists and, especially, their position on de-pathologization, may lead to severe attacks on the part of conservative parliamentarians and general public. This could lead to scaling down trans rights, including access to trans healthcare. It appears that conservative medical specialists, who pathologize trans people, also serve as a shield against political attacks. The fear is that were transgenderism no longer regarded as a medical condition, this protection might suddenly disappear.

One should be cautioned against idealizing the situation of trans healthcare in Russia. It is important to note that while a number of trans-friendly medical services exist in the fields of psychiatry, endocrinology and surgery, they are distributed very unevenly throughout the country. Most are concentrated in Moscow and St. Petersburg, a few in other cities in the European part of Russia, and Western Siberia. Trans people in the whole eastern half of the country often have no competent specialists local to them and need to travel thousands of kilometers at their own expense. Further, it remains an issue that most adequate medical services are provided on a commercial basis. Given the desperate financial situation of most trans people in the country, who suffer from severe transphobia at the workplace, this creates financial barriers to accessing trans-related healthcare. Finally, while there's been a significant growth in the number of medical specialists working in trans-related fields (psychologists, psychiatrists, endocrinologists, gynecologists, surgeons), no similar development can be observed among doctors in other specializations, thus, trans people are subject to transphobic attitudes when accessing general healthcare.

Acknowledgements

I would like to thank Anno Komarov, Egor Burtsev, Eva Steiner and Yael Demedetskaya for the valuable information on medical practices they provided.

References

Belkin, A.I. (2000): Tretij pol. Olimp.

Belkin, A.I. and Karpov, A.S. (1991): Transsexualizm (metodologičeskie rekomendacii po smene pola).

Buxanovskij, A.O. (1994): Transsexualizm: klinika, sistematika, differencial'naâ diagnostika, psixosocial'naâ readaptaciâ i reabilitaciâ. Avtoreferat dissertacii. Rostov-on-Don.

Kalinčenko, S.Y. (2006): Transseksualizm: Vozmožnosti gormonal'noj terapii. Praktičeskaâ medicina.

Kalnberz, V. (2013): Moyo vremya. Medicīnas apgāds.

Kirey-Sitnikova, Y. (2018): How Russian authorities will now process trans people. Available at: https://www.transadvocate.com/how-russian-auth orities-will-now-processes-trans-people_n_22295.htm (Accessed: 04 December 2021).

Kiričenko, K. (2011): Analitičeskaâ zapiska "Položenie transseksual'nyx lûdej v regionax Rossii: Smena dokumentov i dostup k specializirovannoj medicinskoj pomoŝi". Russian LGBT Network.

Kon, I.S. (2008): 80 let odinocestva. Vremâ.

Kozlov, G.I. and Kalinčenko, S.Y. (1995): Slučaj ošibočnoj diagnostiki xroničeskoj nadpočečnikovoj nedostatočnosti u bol'noi mužskim transseksualizmom. In: Problemy endokrinologii, 1, pp. 25-27.

Kučba, N.D.; Istranov, A.L.; Gulâev, I.V.; Vasil'eva, E.E. and Adamân, R.T. (2014): Osložneniâ neovaginoplastiki, sposoby ih korrekcii i profilaktika vozniknoveniâ. In: Andrologiâ i genital'naâ xirurgiâ, 2, pp. 63-69.

Krasnov, V.N. and Gurovič, I.Â. (1999): Kliničeskoe rukovodstvo: Modeli diagnostiki i lečeniâ psihičeskih i povedenčeskih rasstrojstv. Moscow: Moskovskij NII psihiatrii.

Milanov, N.O.; Adamân, R.T. and Kazarân, T.V. (2001): Osložneniâ mikroxirurgičeskoj falloplastiki u transseksualov. In: Annaly plastičeskoj, rekonstruktivnoj i estetičeskoj xirurgii, 1, pp. 62-69.

Mulina, M. (1990): Sergey: Požalujsta, zovite menâ Svetlanoj. Sobesednok, N43.

Popovich, L.; Potapchik, E.; Shishkin, S.; Richardson, E.; Vacroux, A. and Mathivet, B. (2011): Russian Federation: health system review. In: Health Systems in Transition, 13(7).

Healthcare Access of Trans People in Rwanda

Carter Honorée Wolf

Introduction

In 1995, after the period of the genocide, Rwanda started its community health program. Currently, there are approximatively 45,000 CHWs (Community Health Workers) aiming at increasing uptake of essential maternal and child clinical services through education of pregnant persons, promotion of 'healthy' behaviors, and follow-up and linkages to health services. The health system in Rwanda includes 406 health posts, 499 health centers, 44 district hospitals, and four referral hospitals countrywide.

Since its inception, Rwanda's community health program has grown to include an integrated service package that aims at malnutrition screening, treatment of Tuberculosis (TB), prevention of noncommunicable diseases (NCDs), community-based provision of contraceptives, and promotion of 'healthy' behaviors and practices including hygiene, sanitation, family gardens[1]. They likewise play an important role in the fight against HIV, AIDS and malaria.

However, the community health program to the present day fails to address the needs of trans and gender diverse people (TGD). The Rwandan health system does not mention trans and gender diverse people or their needs in documents, nor in any publications. Important aspects of trans healthcare, such as access to mental health services, sexual & reproductive health, HIV services, gender-affirming hormone therapy and gender affirming surgeries are neglected. Trans and gender diverse people's needs, and their access to healthcare were not publicly discussed in the past, nor are they in the present.

---

1   Family gardens are small vegetable gardens owned by families. In my language they are called "akarima k'igikoni".

There is a common misconception that Rwanda does not criminalize homosexuality. While this may be true, it does not reflect the fact that homosexuality is not at all accepted in Rwandan society. In Rwanda, 'homosexuality' refers to everyone who identifies as Lesbian, Gay, Bisexual, Trans, and/or
Queer in the country. As a result, TGD people are forcibly subsumed under
this category. Most TGD people simply choose to not put themselves through
the pain of trying to access healthcare, despite deterioration of their health,
even when they have a health condition that may be fatal. In Rwanda, one has
the right to have sex but not the right to talk about it, especially not about the
health needs and issues that come with an active sexual life.

International Funding of Rwanda's Healthcare System

The Country Operational Plan (COP) 2019 states that in the 2018-2020 Global
Fund funding cycle, Rwanda has been allocated $154 million for HIV pro-
grams, which represents an average of $51.3 million per year. Additionally,
the U.S. President's Emergency Plan for AIDS Relief (PEPFAR) total funding
has fluctuated from $78.5 million in fiscal year (FY) 2017 to $80.9 million in
FY 2018, to $76 million in FY 2019 and to $70 million in FY 2020. Despite internationally supported HIV & AIDS programs, Rwanda's plan to tackle HIV
does not include trans people and there are no indications that it will in the
near future.

Experiences of Trans People in Healthcare Settings

Existing Health programs for trans people are limited to providing services
like HIV tests, distributing lubricants and condoms. However, this approach
completely leaves out mental health, other sexual & reproductive health issues, gender-affirming hormone therapy and gender affirming surgeries.

Rwanda's HIV and AIDS National strategic plan (NSP) 2018-2020 states
that interventions are directed at groups especially susceptible to high transmission of the virus, such as (cis) female sex workers (FSW), (cis) men who
have sex with men (MSM), and serodiscordant couples (SDC). Those more
susceptible groups are offered pre-exposure prophylaxis (PrEP) as a new approach to prevention, along with behavioral and other supportive interventions. The NSP 2018-2020 aims to reduce new HIV infections by 2020 and

strengthen the capacity of health practitioners. Unfortunately, the NSP 2018-2020 does not once mention 'trans people' (RBC n.d.).

In order to obtain HIV services, trans women are forced to participate in programs designed for MSM, since they are excluded from FSW programming. When accessing MSM organizations, trans women are categorized as men who sleep with men, despite the fact that they are women and regardless of their actual sexuality.

Trans men are called 'ibishegabo', which translates to 'a woman who refuses to be a woman and makes herself a man'. Transmasculine people are often obliged to hide their trans identity in order to have access to HIV services. Many anecdotal cases have shown that as soon as someone discloses that they are a trans man, they become a spectacle for the whole health institution they have gone to. Healthcare practitioners start gossiping about having had a 'igishegabo' patient, revealing the person's trans identity for everyone else in that institution. This lack of professionalism by medical staff turns consultation rooms into interrogation rooms and unsafe environments for trans people. Trans patients are ridiculed on the basis of their gender identity and subjected to inappropriate questions about their genitalia. Segregation in health facilities where no health practitioner is at hand to assist trans people is deplorable; the isolation (separation) of gender minorities often based on their identification cards (IDs) and how they physically present and look is used to harass and mistreat trans people asking for medical care. Legal gender recognition, or procedures to change a person's name and gender marker based on a trans identity is not possible in Rwanda. The isolation is successful in health facilities based on how people physically look, dress, walk, their body language and even their voices and their IDs. There are also reported cases of sexual assault experienced by trans people in medical settings in Rwanda.

The discrimination and shaming of trans people inside healthcare institutions by healthcare providers discourages many trans people from seeking medical help. In Rwanda, it is acceptable for doctors to insult and call trans patients names during consultations, and to give advice based on Christian religious beliefs rather than medical research. Some trans people have reported being told by a doctor that if they would accept the 'Christian god', they would be healed of their 'disease'. Many Rwandans, including medical professionals, believe that a trans person may have a demon living inside their body that makes them ill.

It is almost impossible for a trans person to go to a hospital seeking sexual reproductive health services, especially in cases of rape. Frequently, trans men are told that if they were 'really' men they would have been strong enough to protect themselves. Trans women, meanwhile, are reminded about how they have 'gone against the natural law', and that is the reason why they 'deserve to be punished' by being raped. Rape culture is common in Rwandan society, and in the experience of many trans people, rape is justified as a social force which 'corrects' people who do not conform to the gender binary.

> From my personal experience as a Rwandan trans man, before I was able to get an appointment with the endocrinologist, I was obliged to go through psychotherapy, if I wanted to pursue my HRT. I didn't refuse because in my head it was okay, if this would mean I could start the treatment. While doing my sessions I noticed that, not only was I paying from my pocket for the sessions to basically be a teacher to this therapist, but I was actually going through conversion therapy sessions. As I was trying to explain to this person who I am, I would get answers like "but if you changed and lived as God created you, you wouldn't have to go through all the issues you face, you wouldn't feel ashamed of yourself" and other comments like these. The therapy sessions became a way of reminding me that I could be happier, if only I accepted my womanhood and the fact that I am a woman. Each time I sat in that cell I would leave feeling worse than I felt before I left my house. I call it a cell, because now I know it was a sort of indirect prison, where I would take myself each day to listen to this person, telling me all the negative stuff about myself, while on the other side I tried to offer education to them, showed them medical research and facts, and basically taught them how to do their job right. Before I knew it, this therapist set up a meeting with The CHUK (University Teaching Hospital of Kigali) head of department of Mental Health back in 2018 and he gave me two appointments to meet with two different doctors. One doctor was a geneticist to analyze my genes and chromosomes and reproductive parts and the other one was an endocrinologist to 'analyze my gender'. I still did everything I was asked to do, because I hoped after they would see that nothing was wrong with me, I would be prescribed testosterone. Generally speaking, in an 'official' way, gender-affirming hormone therapy (GAHT) is illegal in Rwanda. When I tried to access GAHT in Kigali, a female doctor specialist in endocrinology at one of the biggest hospitals in Rwanda CHUK told me the order of doctors considered GAHT procedure the same as castration. Hence, I should accept that I am a 'beautiful woman' or go seek that treatment outside of Rwanda, because it was impossible in this country. And the reality hit me. I had taken myself to get humiliated, only to then getting humiliated even more!

I remember it was a long hall and I had to cross it 3 times a week for months and I would hear patients seated outside laughing loud, pointing fingers at me, saying slurs like "igishegabo" and "look at how she is dressed and walks like a man". Seated outside of the therapy room cell, patients seated next to me whispered things like "she thinks she is a man, so she dresses like a man" or "yataye umuco" (revolter against the Rwandan culture). The hall was the longest I had to cross. Waiting to be called in was a traumatic event. But I was ready to go through anything if that meant having access to GAHT.

Practitioners in mental health services in Rwanda are largely trained in matters of post-traumatic stress relating to the genocide. They understand gender abuse and rape only to affect cis heterosexuals. LGBTQ people seeking mental health support will usually instead experience some form of conversion therapy. Mental health practitioners will attempt to change you into what they believe you 'should' be.

The Rwandan Health Insurance System

It is said that the poorest citizens in Rwanda are entitled to free health insurance, while the wealthiest pay premiums of $8 per adult monthly. Approximately 90% of the Rwandan population is covered by this scheme. The government system is divided into: *La Rwandaise d'Assurance Maladie* (RAMA) for government civilian employees, MMI (Military Medical Insurance) for the security forces and *Mutuelle de Santé* (MdS), which covers the rest of the general population. Most TGD persons use MdS, which also determines what kind of treatment you will get. Through MdS, one usually does not receive expensive medication. Most drugs prescribed under this coverage are inferior and are prescribed only for the poor. Under the other insurance plans, for those with higher incomes, more expensive and more effective drugs are prescribed.

I have never used Mutuelle de Santé, because using it in hospitals meant being in very long waiting lines, sometimes from the morning until late in the evenings. There was not even a guarantee that one would be treated the same day. Additionally, the attitude and the treatment by reception desk staff and medical practitioners towards trans people is very harsh.

Because of the discriminatory environment in public hospitals, many trans people prefer to attend private clinics. However, not everyone can afford that, and MdS does not cover treatments in private health institutions.

Additional Barriers to Trans Healthcare

Rwandan based non-governmental organizations (NGOs) that claim to work with and for LGBTQ people's access to healthcare services do not understand the particular needs of the trans community and who they are. There is lack of inclusion of trans people in LGBTQ specific projects and a lack of meaningful effort to raise awareness of trans issues. Once a Rwandan based NGO that has a vision for the Right to Health for all people, has answered to questions about health services for trans people by saying: "we have not found yet that trans health is an issue that needs to be addressed". The Rwandan trans community is often dependent on the aforementioned NGOs. However, these organizations rarely or even never seek insight or input from trans people themselves.

TGD persons in Rwanda have very little knowledge about potential health issues that affect their lives, because most have not had access to basic education. Additionally, knowledge about trans health on the internet is rarely accessible. Many Rwandans can't afford to access the internet and, in addition, most resources addressing trans health are in foreign languages that TGD persons in Rwanda don't understand.

The language barrier and the lack of basic education affects the Rwandan trans community in several ways. In surrounding countries and the broader region, trans people are becoming somewhat more widely represented: at conferences, in discussions of health provision, and in political settings. However, one rarely sees Rwandan trans people included. The Rwandan trans community has no access to these spaces, where they might learn from their peers and/or raise awareness about their specific health issues. This exclusion is broadly based on structural barriers; for example, that applications (i.e., for conference registration or conference/meeting scholarships) often need to be filled in languages that Rwandan trans people don't speak. Even if the application process is made more accessible, language barriers at a meeting or conference itself make it difficult to understand what is being talked about in those spaces. Many NGOs, who claim that they represent Rwandan trans people, often have no idea who or what they are representing, since they don't talk to the community. The trans community itself knows best what kind of lives they live and the issues they face every day. Trans people are the experts, even though they can't all speak these foreign languages.

I have been in the presence of western white researchers that come down to Rwanda to speak to the LGBTQ community, but as soon as they realize that we won't be able to understand each other because of the language, they have had the guts to make comments like 'the LGBTQ community in Rwanda is almost non-existent'. What is completely non-existent is English, and speaking it but not my community, and especially their will to want to understand us! Because translators exist or learn our language dammit, we have learnt yours!

This attitude affects the trans community on many levels. There are few resources about the Rwandan LGBTQ community shared online (i.e., Google) and most of them are written by cis, heterosexual people, without having consulted the affected communities, because of the misconception that the affected community has no 'experience' to talk about their own issues. It is a vicious circle, as this information gets shared in international reports, giving out false information and negatively affecting the communities.

This is also made possible because trans people in Rwanda are terrified to speak up. Most Rwandese people are not accustomed to speaking up against injustice, because they have been raised in terror. Expressing personal thoughts can end a person's freedom, land them in jail or even get them killed.

Not speaking a foreign language (i.e., English) shouldn't be the reason why trans people from certain regions are constantly excluded. It shouldn't be an excuse to invite somebody else to speak on their behalf, who is not a member of the community and does not represent them. It shouldn't be the case that trans people have to learn a foreign language to participate in discussions that affect their lives. Likewise, financial barriers such as the high cost of conference registration shouldn't be a reason to prevent trans people from participating in these events.

COVID-19 and Trans Health in Rwanda

COVID-19 has intensified poverty, mental distress, social and government discrimination against trans people in Rwanda.

Trans people already lived in poverty before COVID-19, not having access to basic needs like food and shelter has been a daily struggle. Often employers demand educational diplomas, which is based on the inadequate access to basic education very difficult to provide for most of trans people living in Kigali. Many have been forced or dropped out of schools because of their gender identity and trans people had to leave those environments of physical and mental assaults. During the pandemic, trans people are confronted with the situation of nothing having a possibility to earn money for their daily meals, pay for their rent, medical bills and or even to buy water and soap.

Most trans people in Rwanda do not have running water in their homes. Before the COVID-19 pandemic started, they used to walk miles to get water. But during months of confinement and strict lockdowns, they were even more exposed to police violence, arrests, or even shoot dead, just because they left home to get water. It was a very desperate time for the most vulnerable and many trans people were left without water or soaps for an extended period of time.

Before the COVID-19 pandemic, trans people often gathered among themselves to share some tea, a good laugh or to talk about their daily lives. During the pandemic they were forced into isolation, aggravating the difficult situation in regard to trans people's mental health. Many had no one to talk to, because the majority of trans people in Rwanda do neither have access to internet, nor digital gadgets or to buy phone credit to make calls.

During the pandemic, the government distributed food and other necessities like soap in local areas. However, local leaders who had knowledge about where trans people live, often passed by their homes, refusing to give them food. Their excuse to this segregating behavior against trans people has been that in their opinion trans people deserve bad things happening to them, because trans people are seen as an abomination.

Healthcare providers have used the pandemic as an excuse to refuse care to the trans community. Even trans people with chronic conditions were turned away, based on priorities given to COVID-19 related matters. This situation has increased stigma and discrimination against trans people in the Rwandan medical sector and is causing even a greater burden on the mental health of this community.

To be able to cater for basic needs many trans sex workers in Rwanda still choose to take the risk to meet clients during the pandemic. Because of financial difficulties and not having had access to condoms, lubricants, and medical check-ups, many gave in to the demands of clients for unprotected sex, in exchange for more money.

Additionally, all of 2021 there was a GoFundMe link circulating online and it was meant to raise funds to help LGBTQ people living in Kigali when the

Covid-19 pandemic was raging. However, what was meant to help LGBTQ people in Rwanda, was an initiative to spread lies and humiliate the community.

The fundraising page read as follows (translated to English from Kinyarwanda):

> "After being forced into homosexuality by foreigners who send them money and ask them to teach/convert others into homosexuality, some of the prominent homosexual activists have stopped being homosexuals.
>
> After they stopped being homosexuals, the ones, who promised them miracles, are desperately waiting for them to be struck by extreme poverty/hunger, so they go back to being homosexuals and this has left them with many wounds including many diseases such as being obliged to wear pampers.
>
> Help us lift them up and teach them how to mend for themselves, so the ones (foreigners sending them money) don't find them anymore.
>
> They (the ones who stopped being homosexuals) have a project to travel all around the country (Rwanda) to testify about the dangers and consequences of homosexuality, and to work together for profit making such as making soap.
>
> The projects will cost around 60 million Rwandan Francs ($\sim$ \$58.000). Help the parents and children who are hunted by the devil in these behaviors. Thank you."

Besides struggling with the impact of the pandemic and the general poverty among this population, the local community in Rwanda was confronted with this blatant misrepresentation of LGBTQ people. Those lies portray a false picture of what homosexuality is about, which enforces a negative image about LGBTQ in Rwandan society. Also, the question is raised, who the people on the GoFundMe page photo are and if they are aware of the consequences this has for the LGBTQ community in Rwanda. Although the aim of this project is not entirely clear, it appears that this project aims to raise funds for conversion therapy and clearly shows that Rwandan LGBTQ people need to be protected from such kind of attacks.

Changing the Current Situation

Overcoming these barriers will require attention and effort from people outside of the Rwandan trans community, people who have the power to take the first steps that are needed to include and elevate the voices. This is not an invitation for a takeover. Being a good ally means to educate oneself on trans healthcare needs, to listen to the community, to let the community speak for itself, to let them think for themselves and to let them do their own programming. Give the trans community access to the resources they need, include them in your research, in your publications, and decision making. Don't question them because not having education does not in any case mean that people with education know the trans community's needs better than they do and how to address these needs.

References

Times Reporter (2017): Sponsored: Health Service Delivery in Rwanda grows from strength to strength. In: The News Time, 08 September 2017 [online]. Available at: https://www.newtimes.co.rw/section/read/219527 (Accessed 29 November 2021).

Rwanda Biomedical Centre (RBC, n.d.): Rwanda HIV and AIDS National Strategic Plan 2013-2018. Extension 2018-2020 [Online]. Republic of Rwanda: Ministry of Health. Available at: https://rbc.gov.rw/fileadmin/u ser_upload/stra2019/strategie2019/Rwanda%20Strategic%20Plan%20for %20HIV%20Extended%20to%202020.pdf (Accessed 29 November 2021).

Determinants of Access to Healthcare Among Trans Women in North Central Nigeria

Michael Aondo-verr Kombol

Introduction

Trans women lack visibility and support in Nigerian society. They are often subjected to physical and verbal abuse based on gender. Intolerance perpetrated against trans women in Nigeria is based on many factors, such as religion, culture, legal structures, and political climate. Trans women are not accepted in religious and cultural circles. Most religious groups in Nigeria perceive trans women as an aberration. Furthermore, there are no legal structures in place which protect the rights and existence of trans women. Political discourse in Nigeria is silent about issues relating to trans women. This situation breeds intolerance and violence against trans women. Despite these challenges, trans women still exist and continue surviving in Nigerian society.

All of the above factors, present barriers for trans women in accessing Nigerian health services. This paper aims to investigate how trans women in Nigeria deal with the challenges of their situation and consequently, the extent to which they can access healthcare.

Section I presents an overview of the context of healthcare provision in Nigeria. Section II outlines the state of existing knowledge about the determinants of access to healthcare for trans women in North Central Nigeria. Section III describes the method and findings of the present study. Finally, conclusions and recommendations for future work in this important area are presented.

Section I - the Context of Healthcare Provision in Nigeria

Nigeria is made up of 36 states and the Federal Capital Territory (FCT), Abuja which are grouped into six geo-political zones: North East; North West; North Central; South East; South West and South Kombo. The states which comprise the North Central are: Niger, Kogi, Benue, Plateau, Nassarawa, Kwara and the FCT, Abuja. There are various estimates concerning the population of Nigeria. This is because the last population census was held in 2006 and estimates rely on yearly population growth rate projections. The World Bank (2018) estimates the population of Nigeria to be 195,874,740 people. The Department of Foreign Affairs and Trade, DFAT (2018) finds that there is poor access to healthcare in Nigeria, because demand for public healthcare exceeds supply. Apart from inadequate access to healthcare, the quality of medical service is insufficient. Most Nigerians are unable to afford healthcare. According to The Economist Intelligence Unit (2017), the country is among the five lowest performing countries in the area of equity of access to healthcare. The five lowest performing countries in regard are as follows: Nigeria, Democratic Republic of Congo, Cambodia, Ethiopia and Bangladesh. Each of these countries are populous and economically disadvantaged.

In Nigeria, health services are provided by the government (federal, state, and local); non-governmental organizations; religious organizations; communities and private individuals. Irrespective of the various health service providers, user fees (i.e., immediate cash payment required to access healthcare services) are required from patients to access healthcare services. The percentage of patients who have healthcare insurance is negligible.

Section II - Background to the Study

The healthcare needs of trans women are diverse. They include general healthcare, gender affirming hormone therapy and surgical procedures, as well as psycho-social support. In addition, trans women require regular screening for sexually transmitted infections (STI) and HIV. UNAIDS (2014) estimates that 19% of trans women globally are living with HIV and chances are 49 times higher for trans women to acquire HIV than other adults of reproductive age. Due to this fact, sexual health clinics which focus on key populations in response to the HIV epidemic in Nigeria, often provide services to trans women.

Most of these clinics are trans-friendly and provide treatment for STIs and HIV. However, they do not cover other health needs of trans women.

Several factors determine whether trans women in North Central Nigeria have access to healthcare. They will be explained in this section.

Family Ties and Support

The level of support which trans women in central Nigeria receive from their families vary. In general, trans women are more likely to be supported if their families have higher literacy, greater exposure to information and enlightened social networks, live in an urban area, are of higher socio-economic status, and/or are non-religious.[1] Trans women who have greater support from their families generally have better access to healthcare than those who face hostility and ostracism from their families. Rider et al. (2018) as well as Gower et al. (2017) agree that when families are supportive, patients are protected from discrimination by other people. These patients are protected psychologically because they have family members to turn to when they face discrimination and other forms of maltreatment. By contrast, rejection from family is directly and indirectly detrimental to health.

Level of Education

The level of education that trans women in Nigeria have attained is a significant determinant of access to healthcare. Trans women who have achieved, for example, a bachelor's degree (or beyond), are likely to have better knowledge about healthcare procedures that are available to them. This subset of trans women better understand the benefits, dangers and intricacies of trans affirming healthcare. Furthermore, they are information-seeking, and this often translates to better health outcomes. The opposite is the case when levels of education are low.

Exposure

Urbanization and travel lead to interaction with like-minded people and experience-sharing. This facilitates exposure to trans community, information and support, and increase health seeking behavior among trans women. Latunji and Akinyemi (2018) define health seeking behavior as steps taken by individuals in search of a solution to health problems. Individuals with low health

---

1   Some Christian groups in Nigeria accept trans women more than others.

seeking behavior are more likely to turn to alternative methods, such as self-medication, traditional healers, and patent medicine vendors[2].

Trans women who are exposed to a broader trans community and resources are more likely to seek healthcare beyond services available in Nigeria. Closely related to this phenomenon is the awareness created when trans women are exposed to media, especially the internet and social media. The ability to connect and share information with other trans women has significant implications on accessing healthcare in North Central Nigeria. While health services physically located in Nigeria are often unable to cater to the needs of trans women, if their financial situation allows them, trans women can access some health services over the internet. Online consultations, medication online orders and bookings for medical 'tourism' can all be found in the digital space. The community of trans women in Nigeria is divided between those who are exposed to additional information and access, and those who are not, with the former experiencing generally better health outcomes.

Income Distribution

Income distribution is an important determinant of access to healthcare among trans women in North Central Nigeria. Trans women who have a means of livelihood have better access to healthcare because they can afford to pay for healthcare services when necessary. On the other hand, trans women who do not have viable revenue streams have difficulties in accessing healthcare. With the lack of health insurance for many people in Nigeria, personal income is vital for accessing healthcare. The higher the income of a trans women is, the easier it is to pay for medical services out of pocket.

The World Bank (2015) notes that out of pocket spending accounts for significant expenditure on healthcare in Nigeria, where the public sector spends less than or around 1% of GDP on healthcare. Meanwhile, the World Health Organization (2014) estimates that health accounted for only 8% of budgetary spending in Nigeria. Low overall spending on health services has the additional effect of driving prices for health services up, in contrast to countries with systems of universal health insurance.

---

2   In Nigeria, *Patent Medicine Vendors* are government approved shops which sell medicines to members of the public often without prescriptions.

Quality and Quantity of Healthcare

Trans women's perceptions about the quality of healthcare available also affect the possibilities of access. Negative perceptions of the healthcare system are rife, and well founded. Most health services do not address the needs of trans women with regard to hormonal treatments, sexually transmitted infections, cosmetic procedures, gender affirmation surgeries, etc. Due to a significant lack of these services in the Nigerian healthcare system, trans women often resort to self-medication, with advice from other trans women within their social circles. Trans women with low economic resources turn to alternative medicine (i.e., traditional medicine) and untrained personnel. Often these untrained personnel pretend to be medical professionals for the treatment of sexually transmitted infections, like chlamydia, gonorrhea, syphilis, genital warts, etc. Also, some health facilities pose significant risk to patients due to unsafe practices. Alsulami, Conroy and Choonara (2013: 995-1008) state that unsafe care is characterized by wrong prescriptions, over-dosage and poor hospital hygiene, which often results in the death and disability of patients. Perceived notions of unsafe care circulating in social networks among trans women in decrease these women's willingness to access the available care. They avoid these health facilities and instead attempt to refer themselves to facilities which they perceive as safe and efficient.

Lack of Expertise in Trans Medicine

Trans women are not officially recognized in Nigerian society. Additionally, most medical professionals lack the medical expertise to treat the health needs of trans women. One of these needs is the prescription of gender affirming hormone therapy. Since few medical professionals in Nigeria are competent or willing to provide this kind of care, many trans women rely on the experiences of other community members and engage in self-medication. Nigeria does not have a strict system of medical prescriptions; therefore, patients are able to purchase medicine over the counter without a prescription. Self-medication occurs when trans women treat medical conditions on their own, without the supervision of a health professionals. The practice of medically unsupervised self-medication may lead to undesired outcomes. Sanchez, Sanchez and Danoff (2009) reiterate that doctors' lack of expertise in trans medicine is a major impediment to healthcare access. Trans women are rightfully hesitant to consult a doctor who may not understand their issues due to lack of expertise. Unger (2015) as well as Vance, Halpern-Felsher and Rosenthal (2015) assert that expertise in trans medicine is lacking because it is not taught in conventional medical curricula. These factors make practitioners in general medicine ignorant when it comes to diagnosis and treatment of health conditions faced by trans women. Furthermore, Vance, Halpern-Felsher and Rosenthal (2015) add that most doctors are unable or unwilling to undertake trans specific procedures such as implants (breast, buttock and cheek), and they are unlikely to understand that trans women face a higher risk of cardiovascular diseases, cancer, depression/anxiety and alcohol/substance use. All of these factors mean that trans women are less willing to consult with doctors regarding their health needs, and when they do, the quality of care that they receive is low.

Attitude of Health Professionals in Nigeria
The attitude of health professionals in Nigerian hospitals also determines the access to healthcare for trans women. Unfortunately, Nigeria does not have legislation which protect trans women from discrimination perpetrated by doctors, nurses, ward attendants and other healthcare professionals. Owing to this, trans women in central Nigeria report unsavory practices from healthcare professionals such as: physical and verbal abuse, extra waiting times, improper/refusal of care, invasion of privacy, verbal abuse, etc. These health professionals include: doctors, nurses, lab technicians, para-medical staff, ward attendants, etc. When health professionals in Nigerian hospitals do not treat trans women with respect, trans women are unlikely to use such health services in the future.

Given this discriminatory environment in medical settings, community friendly clinics (i.e., community friendly drop-in centers and One Stop Shops, OSS) are on the rise in Nigeria. However, these friendly services are restricted to STI and HIV treatment. When they need other medical care, trans women must turn to general medical services and they are again exposed to discrimination.

Criminalization
According to Carroll and Mendos (2017), Nigeria is among the 57 countries of the world where it is a crime to be trans. Significant numbers of trans women in Nigeria are afraid of coming out to receive healthcare because they can be charged with impersonation by the police, which is a criminal offence in Nigeria (Carroll and Mendos, 2017). Makofane et al. (2012) establish a rela-

tionship between criminalization of trans women and the upward incidence of HIV among this key population. They conclude that decriminalizing trans identity will improve acceptance in society, increase access to healthcare and address the health risks associated with spread of HIV within this community. Governments of countries where being trans is criminalized need to emulate other progressive nations where trans people are legal and accepted. This is a vital precondition for improving the health of the trans community.

The Role of Traditional Medicine

Alongside Western medicine, traditional medicine is widely practiced in Nigeria. In comparison to orthodox (mainstream) medicine, traditional medicine is relatively affordable, within reach and locally available. Skills and resources (i.e., roots, seeds, herbs, potions, etc.,) are passed on from one generation to another and practitioners are found in many communities around Nigeria. The World Health Organization refers to traditional medicine as Traditional, Complementary and Alternative Medicine (TCAM)[3].

The medicines in TCAM are often herbal and unique to communities and ethnic groups all over Nigeria. Apart from the use of herbs, Adinma, Azuike and Okafor-Udah (2015) note that some TCAM approaches in Nigeria incorporate faith-based methods with the use of spirituality and prayer. The cost of TCAM is relative to the ailment being treated and the practitioners providing the service. Notions of the efficacy and cost effectiveness of TCAM fuel its popularity among some trans women. Thus, some trans women prefer TCAM over mainstream healthcare. While this is not inherently problematic, in some cases accessing TCAM can reduce propensity to access mainstream medicine. This has implications, for example, for the spread of HIV, because patients who are not accessing mainstream HIV medications are more likely to have detectable viral loads and spread HIV to others (Elsinger, Dieffenbach and Fauci (2019).

---

3   In Nigeria, TCAM are indigenous healthcare practices which exist outside the mainstream health system.

Section III – the Present Study

Purpose of the Study

This study aimed to further investigate the above-identified determinants of access to healthcare among trans women in North Central Nigeria. Participants were asked about their level of education and type of employment, their degree of exposure to information on trans health issues, whether they had health insurance or paid out of pocket for healthcare, the extent of family support and whether families were involved in paying for healthcare. In this way, the study identified whether trans women in North Central Nigeria had access to mainstream healthcare and investigated reasons why or why not. For those who did not have access to mainstream healthcare, the study identified the alternatives that they turned to and why.

Method

The study employed a survey (qualitative and quantitative) which used an open-ended questionnaire to enable respondents express themselves freely without the restriction of close ended questions. Copies of the questionnaire were administered to trans women in North Central Nigeria with the use of research assistants. The studied population was trans women in the following states (i.e., regions) of North Central Nigeria: Plateau, Benue, Niger, Nassarawa, Kwara, Kogi, and the Federal Capital Territory (FCT) Abuja. These five states were selected for the study due to the presence of community friendly (i.e., trusted) health centers in these areas, which provide HIV and STI services to trans women. The research assistants were indigenous to the study locations. They were ethnically competent and understood the terrain. In each of these locations, one research assistant facilitated data collection, while in Abuja, there were two research assistants assigned to this task due to the size of the city. Data collection was anonymous due to legal restrictions and the respondents were assured of confidentiality. Toward the end, identifiers such as names, addresses and telephone numbers of the respondents were erased. Due to the hard-to-reach nature of study population, the research assistants employed a snowballing referral system, in which the initial trans women selected for the study (who were identified in community friendly health centers) suggested other prospective respondents. Participation in the study was voluntary. Some copies of the questionnaire were orally administered to respondents who were not literate or had linguistic challenges due to preference of an ethnic Nigerian language. The ethnic competence and linguistic ability of the research assistants ensured that this limitation was overcome.

Findings

The study had 124 respondents spread across locations in Nigeria

Table I: Geographical Distribution of Respondents

s/n	Location	Respondents	Percentage
1	FCT/Abuja	34	27.4%
2	Benue	20	16.1
3	**Nassarawa**	**26**	**20.9**
4	Niger	23	18.6
5	Plateau	21	17
	Total	124	100

The FCT/Abuja had the highest number of respondents because it is cosmopolitan and because there were two research assistants working in the area **identifying respondents for the study.**

Table II: Age of Respondents

s/n	Age Brackets	Respondents	Percentage
1	21-25	25	20.2
2	26-30	31	25
3	**31-35**	**28**	**22.6**
4	36-40	27	21.8
5	Over 40 years	13	10.4
	Total	124	100

The respondents of the study were predominantly younger. The study was unable to reach large numbers of trans women who are older, especially those who are over 40 years of age. This does not necessarily mean that they do not exist in Nigeria.

Table III: Levels of Education

s/n	Education	Respondent	Percentage
1	Tertiary	21	16.9
2	Trade Qualifications	36	29
3	**Secondary School**	**26**	**21**
4	Primary School	33	26.6
5	No Formal Education	8	6.5
	Total	124	100

A significant percentage of respondents (29%) had trade qualifications such as: hair dressing, nail artistry, make-up, event planning, interior decorating, dress making, catering, etc.

Table IV: Employment

s/n	Employment	Respondent	Percentage
1	Self Employed	109	87.9
2	Formal Employment	15	12.1
	Total	**124**	**100**

While a significant number of respondents are self-employed in the private sector others are employed in formal settings with an identified employer. Respondents indicated that self-employment among trans women in Nigeria enables them escape criticism and discrimination from employers and colleagues in formal work settings. With self-employment, they are masters of their own businesses and are not accountable to anyone.

None of the respondents in the study had health insurance, including those respondents in formal work settings. Thus, they have to pay for healthcare out of pocket. This places a financial burden on the respondents. In addition, only 18 respondents (14.5%) received support from their families in order to pay healthcare bills. The lack of family support is a significant barrier, which affects access to healthcare among the remaining 106 (85.5%) respondents. These respondents indicated that they did not receive any support from families towards healthcare costs because their relatives did not approve of their gender expression. Families in Nigeria are often close knit and it is normal to contribute towards healthcare costs of family members. However, this is not the case for these respondents whose families consider the lives they live as an aberration.

Levels of education and exposure to information among respondents in the study had significant consequences vis-à-vis awareness of trans health issues. As indicated earlier, 8 (6.5%) of the respondents had no school education. However, all the respondents indicated that they have access to information about trans topics and issues from informal social networks of trans women, and that this significantly affects their health seeking behavior. 104 respondents (83.8%) indicated that access to information via informal social networks among trans women is the most significant source of information on trans health issues. Information sharing among the respondents is an important channel of transmission for health-related information that in turn influences health seeking behavior of the respondents. In spite of the willingness of participants to seek to access healthcare, the rate of access to mainstream health services is low. 98 respondents (79%) indicated that they self-medicate, buy from patent medicine vendors or access TCAM and that these are the best options available to them considering their circumstances. Low propensity to access mainstream healthcare is based on the fear of facing stigma and discrimination from healthcare workers and perceived lack of trans-specific expertise in healthcare providers. Both significantly affect quality and quantity of healthcare for trans women. These factors were identified by many respondents as barriers to accessing mainstream healthcare.

From the study population, 108 respondents (87%) indicated that they are unable to access mainstream healthcare because they are unable to pay, especially for hormone therapy and surgeries. Thus, they resort to cheaper alternatives such as self-medication, patent medicine vendors and TCAM. Lower or unreliable income, due to the high rate of self-employment, leads to decreased inability to pay for health insurance or for mainstream healthcare. In some instances, respondents also reported preferring TCAM over mainstream healthcare because they believed it would be more effective; for example, in the prevention or treatment of STIs. All the respondents agreed that criminalization fuels fear of being reported by healthcare providers, and that hostile attitudes by mainstream doctors further reduce propensity to access these services.

Conclusion and Recommendations

Access to healthcare is vital in the lives of trans women in Nigeria. This community requires transition-related care, general medical care and also specialist care for HIV prevention and treatment. Factors that can limit trans women's access to care include: low family support, low levels of education, low income, low quality of available care, poor expertise and hostile attitudes among health professionals, as well as previous experiences of stigma and discrimination. Many of these factors are inter-related and lead to undesired outcomes, including over-reliance by trans women on alternative practices such as self-medication and TCAM.

This situation requires action from relevant stakeholders in the healthcare system, especially funders and program implementers. These establishments should consider the implementation of unique models of healthcare provision that consider the predicament of trans women in Nigeria. This can include (but may not be limited to) broadening the current approach of community friendly centers, so that as well as HIV and STI testing and treatment, these centers can provide other essential medical services to trans women. These facilities are already considered safe points of access to healthcare by many trans women and could therefore play an important role in broadening the variety of health services that trans women can access.

There is an urgent need for community-inclusive research by health services about trans women in Nigeria. For example, TCAM can be cost effective and accessible form of healthcare for trans women, but there is a need for the efficacy of particular treatments to be scientifically verified. Research and its subsequent application are needed to interrogate beneficial intersections between the healthcare needs of trans women in Nigeria and TCAM practices.

In the long run, it will be necessary to set up legal structures in Nigeria modelled on the example of other progressive countries where trans women are accepted and protected by law. This would reduce the stigma and discrimination that trans women face and remove some of the barriers that they encounter as they access healthcare. The decriminalization of trans identity may pave way for legal gender recognition in Nigeria and acceptance of trans people. It is vitally necessary to advocate for legal and cultural change so that trans people are no longer perceived as an aberration in Nigerian society, but rather as a unique population with health needs that should be catered for. Trans people, like all citizens, have a right to healthcare in order to realize their full potential in society.

References

Aaron, O. (2016): Growing Recognition of Transgender Health. In: Bulletin of the World Health Organization, 94, pp. 790-791.

Adinma, E.; Azuike, E. and Okafor-Udah, C. (2015): Pattern and practice of complementary and alternative medication amongst patients in a tertiary hospital in Nigeria. In: European Journal of Preventive Medicine, 3, pp. 44–48.

Alsulami, Z.; Conroy, S. and Choonara, I. (2013): Medication errors in the Middle East Countries: A systematic review of the literature. In: European Journal of Clinical Pharmacology, 69(4), pp. 995-1008.

Asuzu, C.C.; Elumelu-Kupoluyi, T.; Asuzu, M.C.; Campbell, O.B.; Akin-Odayne, E.O. and Lounsbury, D. (2017): A pilot study of cancer patients' use of traditional healers in the Radiotherapy Department, University College Hospital, Ibadan, Nigeria. In: Psychooncology, 26(3), pp. 369-376.

Asscherman, H.; Giltay, E.J.; Megens, J.A.; Pim de Ronde, W.; Van Trotsenburg, M.A.A. and Gooren, L.J. (2011): A long-term follow-up of mortality in transsexuals receiving treatment with cross-sex hormones. In: European Journal of Endocrinology, 164(4), pp. 635-642.

Babajide, K.; Crowell T.A.; Nowak, R.G.; Adebajo, S.; Peel, S.; Gaydos, C.A.; Rodriguez-Hart, C.; Baral, S.D.; Walsh, M.J.; Njoku, O.S.; Odeyemi, S.; Ngo-Ndomb, T.; Blattner, W.A.; Robb, M.L.; Charurat, M.E. and Ake, J. (2016): High prevalence of HIV, chlamydia and gonorrhoea among men who have sex with men and transgender women attending trusted community centres in Abuja and Lagos, Nigeria. In: Journal of the International AIDS Society, 19, p. 21270.

Baral, S.D.; Poteat, T.; Stromdahl, S.; Wirtz, A.; Guadamuz, TE. and Beyrer, C. (2013) Worldwide burden of HIV in transgender women: a systematic review and meta-analysis. In: Lancet Infect Dis, 13(3), pp. 214-222.

Becasen, J.S.; Denard, C.L.; Mullins, M.M.; Higa, D.H. and Sipe, T.A. (2018): Estimating the prevalence of HIV and sexual behaviors among the US transgender population: a systematic review and meta-analysis, 2006-2017. In: Am J Public Health, 109(1), pp. e1–e8.

British Medical Association and the Commonwealth Medical Trust (BMA and COMMAT, 2007): The Right to Health: A tool kit for health professionals. London: BMA.

Carroll, A. and Mendos, L.R. (2017): State Sponsored Homophobia 2017: A world survey of sexual orientation laws: criminalisation, protection and recognition (12th ed.). Geneva: ILGA.

Celkis, P. and Venckiene, E. (2011): Concept of the Right to health. In: Jurisprudence, 18(1), pp. 269-286.

Department of Foreign Affairs and Trade (DFAT, 2018): DFAT Country Information Report Nigeria [online]. Sydney: Australian Government. Available at: https://www.dfat.gov.au/sites/default/files/country-information -report-nigeria.pdf (Accessed 22 November 2021).

Eisinger, R.W.; Dieffenbach, C.W. and Fauci, A.S. (2019): HIV Viral Load and Transmissibility of HIV Infection: Undetectable Equals Untransmittable. In: Journal of the American Medical Association JAMA, 321(5), pp. 451-452.

Gerwen, O.V.; Munzy, C.; Austin, E.; Musgrove, K. and Jani, A. (2019): Prevalence of STIs and HIV in transgender women and men: a systematic review. In: Sexually Transmitted Infections, 95, p. A335.

Global Library of Women's Medicine (2016): Integrated Competencies for Medical Practice [online]. Available at: https://www.glowm.com/integra ted-competencies (Accessed 22 November 2021).

Gower, A.L.; Forster, M.; Gloppen, K.; Johnson, A. Z.; Eisenberg, M.E.; Connett, J.E. and Borowsky, I.W. (2018): School practices to foster LGBT supportive climate: associations with adolescent bullying involvement. In: Prev Sci, 19(6), pp. 813-821.

Guadamuz, T.E.; Wimonsate, W.; Varangrat, A.; Phanuphak, P.; Jommaroeng, R.; McNicholl, J.M.; Mock, P.A.; Tappero, J.W. and Van Griensven, F. (2011): HIV prevalence, risk behavior, hormone use and surgical history among transgender persons in Thailand. In: AIDS Behav., 15, pp. 650–658.

Haas, A.P.; Rodgers, P.L. and Herman, J.L. (2014): Suicide Attempts among Transgender and Gender Non-Conforming Adults: Findings of the National Transgender Discrimination Survey [online]. New York and Los Angeles: American Foundation for Suicide Prevention and The Williams Institute. Available at: https://escholarship.org/uc/item/8xg8061f (Accessed 22 November 2021).

Herbst, J.H.; Jacobs, E.D.; Finlayson, T.J.; McKleroy, V.S.; Neumann, M.S. and Crepaz, N. (2008): Estimating HIV prevalence and risk behaviors of transgender persons in the United States: a systematic review. In: AIDS Behav., 12, pp. 1–17.

James, P.B.; Wardle, J.; Steel, A.; and Adams, J. (2018): Traditional, complementary and alternative medicine use in Sub Saharan Africa: a systematic review. In: BMJ Glob Health, 3(5), p. 000895.

James, S.E.; Herman, J.L.; Rankin, S.; Keisling, M.; Mottet, L. and Anafi, M. (2016): The Report of the 2015 U.S. Transgender Survey [online]. Washington, D.C.: National Center for Transgender Equality. Available at: https://transequality.org/sites/default/files/docs/usts/USTS-Full-Report-Dec17.pdf (Accessed 22 November 2021).

King, M.; Semlyen, J.; Tai, S.S.; Killaspy, H.; Osborn, D.; Popelyuk, D. and Nazareth, I. (2008): A systematic review of mental disorder, suicide, and deliberate self-harm in lesbian, gay and bisexual people. In: BMC Psychiatry, 8(70), pp. 1-17.

Lagarde, M. and Palmer, N. (2011): The impact of user fees on access to health services in low- and middle-income countries. In: The Cochrane Database of Systematic Reviews, 4, p. CD009094.

Latunji, O.O. and Akinyemi, O.O. (2018): Factors Influencing Health Seeking Behaviour Among Civil Servants in Ibadan, Nigeria. In: Annals of Ibadan Postgraduate Medicine, 16(1), pp. 52–60.

Makofane, K.; Gueboguo, C.; Lyons, D. and Sandfort, T. (2012): Men who have sex with men inadequately addressed in African AIDS National Strategic Plans. In: Global Public Health, 8(2), pp. 129-143.

National Bureau of Statistics (NBS, 2018): Demographic Statistics Bulletin. Abuja: NBS.

Nemoto, T.; Iwamoto, M.; Perngparn, U.; Areesantichai, C.; Kamitani, E. and Sakata, M. (2012): HIV-related risk behaviors among kathoey (male-to-female transgender) sex workers in Bangkok, Thailand. In: AIDS Care, 24, pp. 210–219.

Onifade, A.A.; Ajeigbe, K.O.; Omotosho, I.O.; Rahamon, S.K. and Oladeinde, B.H. (2013): Attitude of HIV patients to herbal remedy for HIV infection in Nigeria. In: Niger Journal of Physiological Science, 28, pp. 109–112.

Operario, D.; Nemoto, T.; Iwamoto, M. and Moore, T. (2011): Unprotected sexual behavior and HIV risk in the context of primary partnerships for transgender women. In: AIDS Behav., 15, pp. 674–682.

Peters, D.H.; Garg, A.; Bloom, G.; Walker, D.G.; Brieger, W.R. and Hafizur Rahman, M. (2008): Poverty and access to healthcare in developing countries. In: Ann NY Acad Sci, 1136(1), pp. 161-171.

Rider, G.N.; McMorris, B.J.; Gower, A.L.; Coleman, E. and Eisenberg, M.E. (2018): Health and Care Utilization of Transgender and Gender Non-conforming Youth: A Population-Based Study. In: Pediatrics 141(3), p. e20171683.

Sanchez, N.F.; Sanchez, J.P. and Danoff, A. (2009): Health care utilization, barriers to care, and hormone usage among male-to-female transgender persons in New York City. In: Am J Public Health, 99(4), pp. 713– 719.

The Economist Intelligence Unit (2017): Global Access to Health Care: Building Sustainable Health Systems [online]. Available at: https://impact.econom ist.com/perspectives/perspectives/sites/default/files/Globalaccesstohealt hcare-3.pdf (Accessed 22 November 2021).

The Free Dictionary by Farlex (2018): Health Care [online]. Available at: https: //www.thefreedictionary.com/health+care (Accessed 22 November 2021).

The Joint United Nations Programme on HIV/AIDS (UNAIDS, 2014): Trans-gender People [online]. In: UNAIDS (2014): The Gap Report. Geneva: UNAIDS, pp. 214-228. Available at: https://www.unaids.org/sites/defaul t/files/media_asset/UNAIDS_Gap_report_en.pdf (Accessed 22 November 2021).

The World Bank (2015): Current Health expenditure (% of GDP) [online]. Available at: https://data.worldbank.org/indicator/SH.XPD.CHEX.GD.Z S (Accessed 22 November 2021).

The World Bank (2018): Nigeria [online]. Available at: https://data.worldbank .org/country/NG (Accessed 22 November 2021).

The World Bank (2019): The World Bank in Nigeria. Overview [online]. Available at: https://www.worldbank.org/en/country/nigeria/overview (Accessed 22 November 2021).

Unger, C.A. (2012): Care of the transgender patient: A survey of gynecologists' current knowledge and practice. In: Journal of Women's Health, 26, pp. 114–118.

United Nations (2015): Universal Declaration of Human Rights [online]. Available at: https://www.un.org/en/udhrbook/pdf/udhr_booklet_en_web.pdf (Accessed 22 November 2021).

Vaisvila, A. (2009): Theory of Law. Vilnius: Justitia.

Vance, S.R.; Halpern-Felsher, B.L. and Rosenthal, S.M. (2015): Health care providers' comfort with and barriers to care of transgender youth. In: Journal of Adolescent Health, 56, pp. 251–253.

Verster, A. (2016): Growing Recognition of Transgender Health. In: Bulletin of the World Health Organization, 94, pp. 790-791.

Winter, S.; Diamond, M.; Green, J.; Karasic, D.; Reed, T.; Whittle, S. and Wylie, K. (2016): Transgender people: Health at the margins of society. In: The Lancet, 388(10041), pp. 390-400.

World Health Organization (WHO, 2011): Prevention and Treatment of HIV and Other Sexually Transmitted Infections Among Men Who Have Sex with Men and Transgender People: Recommendations for a public health approach [online]. Available at: http://apps.who.int/iris/bitstream/handl e/10665/44619/9789241501750_eng.pdf;jsessionid=83B4B92629034454B996 C97B76B8C658?sequence=1 (Accessed 22 November 2021).

World Health Organization (WHO, 2014): WHO Traditional Medicine Strategy 2014-2023 [online]. Available at: https://apps.who.int/iris/bitstream/hand le/10665/92455/9789241506090_eng.pdf (Accessed 22 November 2021).

World Health Organization (WHO, 1946): Constitution of the World Health Organization. [online]. Available at: https://treaties.un.org/doc/Treaties /1948/04/19480407%2010-51%20PM/Ch_IX_01p.pdf (Accessed 29 January 2022).

Access to Gender-Affirming Care in South Africa – A Landscape in Transition

Elma De Vries & Chris/tine McLachlan

Until recently, access to gender-affirming care in South Africa has been very difficult, especially in the public health sector. Not only does this have an impact on gender affirming possibilities for trans and gender diverse (TGD) people, but it also has an impact on TGD people's mental health. This landscape is gradually transforming, with great developments in improved access to care as well as new models of care.

Health Disparities

Compared to cisgender people, TGD people internationally experience significant health disparities and an increased burden of disease (Reisner et al. 2016). Specific health risks include increased risk of mental health challenges, violence and victimization, substance use, and a disproportionately high prevalence of the Human Immunodeficiency Virus (HIV), as evidenced by South African research which will be discussed below.

A recent survey on the realities of violence, mental health and access to healthcare related to Sexual orientation, Gender Identity and Expression (SOGIE) found alarming rates of mental health challenges amongst South African TGD respondents: depression as measured with the CES-D 10 (63%), anxiety as measured with the GAD-7 (39%) and suicide attempts in the past year (16%) (Müller, Daskilewicz and the Southern and East African Research Collective on Health 2019).[1] Experience of sexual violence in the past year was reported

---

1   CES-D 10 is Centre for Epidemiological Studies Depression Scale (CES-D-10), a validated screening tool. GAD-7 is Generalized Anxiety Disorder 7-item scale, a validated screening tool. AUDIT is Alcohol Use Disorders Identification Test, a 10-item screen-

by 35% of trans women and 28% of trans men. Alcohol use that was classified as hazardous/harmful/dependence with the AUDIT instrument, was reported in 46%, with drug use that was classified as harmful/dependence with the DU-DIT instrument in 25% of respondents. A Cape Town study found that 57% of gender non-conforming participants (who identified as female or 'transgender') had tested HIV positive compared to 31% of the male-identifying participants (Jobson et al. 2018). Some trans women in South Africa turn to commercial sex work for survival (Samudzi and Mannell 2016). A study of South African sex workers found that the trans women were 2.4 times more likely than cis female respondents to have unprotected sex, which increases HIV risk (Richter et al. 2013). At the time that the data for this study was collected (2010), public health messaging about HIV in South Africa was mostly heteronormative, with very limited public health interventions focusing on trans sex workers.

Legal and Policy Framework in South Africa

The Bill of Rights in the South African Constitution guarantees every citizen rights regardless of one's "race, gender, sex, [...] sexual orientation [or] age"; the respect and protection of their inherent dignity; the right to life; freedom and security of their person including protection from inhumane and degrading treatment; and the preservation of "bodily and psychological integrity," including sovereignty in decisions regarding reproduction and control over the body (Hatchard 1994). The Promotion of Equality and Prevention of Unfair Discrimination Act of 2000 protects individuals on the basis of gender, while explicitly differentiating between gender and sex (Republic of South Africa 2000).

Section 27 of the South African constitution states that everyone has the right to have access to healthcare services, including reproductive healthcare (Hatchard 1994). It further declares that the state must take reasonable legislative and other measures, within its available resources, to achieve the progressive realization of each of these rights.

Before 2003, it was not possible for a trans person to change their gender marker in their identity document in South Africa. This changed with the Al-

---

ing tool developed by the WHO. DUDIT is Drug Use Disorders Identification Test, an 11-item validated screening tool.

teration of Sex Description and Sex Status Act 49 of 2003, which prescribes a process requiring two medical reports stating that "gender reassignment" (the wording in the Act) has taken place (Republic of South Africa 2003). While on paper the law says it is possible to change one's gender marker, the implementation of Act 49 has been very inconsistent (Hamblin and Nduna 2013; Klein 2012). A Legal Resource Centre report describes the unjust delayed and improper processing of applications, as well as unfair and baseless rejections, and argues that the implementation issues of the Act amount to unjust administration and violate the right to equality, dignity, privacy and just administration (Mudarikwa, May and Martens 2017).

In South African healthcare, recent years have brought a shift to include LGBT health in healthcare policy recommendations. Trans people were identified as one of the most-at-risk populations in the 2012–2016 National Strategic Plan for HIV, STIs and TB (SANAC 2012). In the subsequent 2017-2022 Strategic Plan, the language changed from "most-at-risk populations" to "key populations", for HIV and STIs, using the UNAIDS and WHO definitions. This identifies trans people as one of the key populations. This document sets the goal of: "Reach[ing] all key and vulnerable populations with customised and targeted intervention services" (SANAC 2017). In December 2019, the Essential Medicine List of the Department of Health for the first time included hormones specifically for treatment of 'gender dysphoria' (NEMLC 2019).

Despite progressive legislation, conservative social attitudes persist in South African society, including in healthcare settings. In a recent representative population survey, 66% of South Africans reported that they are 'disgusted' by gender non-conformity (Gabriel 2016). This survey estimated that over the previous 12 months, around half a million (450,000) South Africans have physically harmed people that they believed to be women whom they deemed to be dressing or behaving in ways that were too masculine. Likewise, 240,000 have assaulted people who they believed to be men, whom they deemed to be dressing or behaving in ways that were too feminine. Approximately 700,000 South Africans verbally abused (shouted at or teased) gender non-conforming people.

Experiences of TGD Persons in Accessing Care in South Africa

While some of the studies report on sexual as well as gender minorities, there is a small but growing body of evidence specifically on trans experiences. In a South African study of queer people's experiences, participants reported feeling keenly aware that the physical spaces of the healthcare facilities that they had visited overwhelmingly suggested that they were by and for heterosexual and gender-normative people (Meer and Müller 2017). Participants pointed out that the more non-normative one appears, the greater the vulnerability to homo- and transphobia is. This is of particular relevance to trans persons who do not fit into the binary expression of gender (Meer and Müller 2017). A qualitative study analyzed the experiences of 16 LGBT health service users accessing South African public sector healthcare (Müller 2017). This study found that all participants reported experiences of discrimination by healthcare providers based on their sexual orientation and/or gender identity, such as disrespectful treatment, verbal harassment and religious judgment. A recurrent theme in this study was delayed health-seeking behavior, or the avoidance of health facilities by people who identify as LGBT. Barriers to accessing care include fear of experiencing discrimination, homophobia, or secondary victimization, as well as with an understanding that public facilities often do not or cannot provide care for LGBT-specific health concerns. As a result of health rights violations that they had either experienced themselves, or had heard about from friends and peers, many participants expressed their fear of judgement and discrimination when accessing public health facilities. This resonates with the minority stress model that describes three processes, where the second process described is negative expectations that delay health seeking behavior and also exacerbate the impact of discrimination when it occurs (Hendricks and Testa 2012).

A case study of barriers faced by trans persons when accessing health services in Gauteng reported condescending attitudes by health workers as well as an observation that staff members were not adequately equipped with the necessary skills to offer adequate health services to trans people (Nkoana and Nduna 2012). A qualitative study done in Gauteng and Mpumalanga found that respondents experienced discrimination in the South African medical system due to the wide prevalence of a rigid understanding of gender and sexuality (Husakouskaya 2013).

A key survey on trans people's access to sexual health services in South Africa reported that many of the participants experienced health workers as discriminatory and hostile (Stevens 2012). This survey described multiple layers of discrimination in South African healthcare facilities, ranging from verbal abuse to denial of care. It is important to note that such discrimination is not only perpetrated by individual healthcare providers. Rather, it is a structural problem deeply rooted in the health system itself (Müller 2016). The health system is experienced as heteronormative and cis-normative with little understanding of non-conforming sexualities and gender identities.

Qualitative studies in South Africa have described the negative experiences of trans people when trying to access healthcare. A study of 17 young trans persons in South Africa described discriminatory treatment in the health sector, especially for trans persons who feel they are not easily 'read' according to their gender identity (Sanger 2014). In the Western Cape a study of 10 trans women described an imbalance in the power relationship between healthcare practitioners and trans women, with experiences of ill-treatment and breaches of confidentiality (Newman-Valentine and Duma 2014). In Kwazulu-Natal, participants reported that when they asked for gender-affirming services, they were met with confusion from healthcare workers who were unable to offer care, advice or appropriate referral (Luvuno, Ncama, and Mchunu 2019). Participants reported experiences of violation of bodily privacy through healthcare worker voyeurism and deliberate exposure of the trans-status of the patient to other patients. Their experience was that all health problems were turned into problems concerning gender identity, even if the patient was seeking care for a different, unrelated reason, with one participant reporting that even though she went to the clinic for a broken bone, she was made to undress (ibid.).

A survey on the realities of violence, mental health and access to healthcare related to SOGIE reported disturbing findings regarding access to healthcare (Müller, Daskilewicz and the Southern and East African Research Collective on Health 2019). Of the South African TGD respondents, 48% reported having been called names or insulted in a health facility because of their gender identity and 39% reported that they had been denied healthcare because of their gender identity (ibid.).

Landscape in Transition

South Africa has a quadruple burden of disease, that has been described as colliding of epidemics: HIV and tuberculosis; chronic illness and mental health; injury and violence; and maternal, neonatal, and child health (Mayosi et al. 2012). In this context, gender-affirming care has not been regarded as a high priority. Access to gender-affirming care is severely limited and unequal within South Africa, with a 2017 publication reporting access to care in public hospitals in only 4 of the 9 provinces (Spencer, Meer and Müller 2017). The researchers found that while a small minority of healthcare providers offer gender affirming care, this is almost exclusively on their own initiative and is usually unsupported by wider structures and institutions. A specific concern is the limited access to gender-affirming surgery, with waiting lists of 15-20 years (Wilson et al. 2014). Of the South African TGD participants in the survey on the realities of violence, mental health and access to healthcare related to SOGIE (Müller, Daskilewicz and the Southern and East African Research Collective on Health 2019), only 28% used hormones. Participants were significantly more likely to report using hormones if they had medical aid or health insurance ($p < .05$).

Medical aids (health insurance) in South Africa do not generally fund gender-affirming care, although the case for 'medical necessity' has convincingly been argued by the Legal Resource Centre (Mudarikwa, May and Martens 2017). Gender affirming private healthcare is not easily accessible in South Africa, due to unaffordability for most people (Koch et al. 2019).

The landscape is gradually changing with more public hospitals and general practitioners providing access to hormones, and a project to pilot four primary care clinics for trans people to access HIV prevention and treatment as well as hormones by WITS RHI. Not-for-profit organizations have advocated for improved access to care and have provided training for health professionals in gender-affirming care. The argument has been made for inclusion of gender-affirming care in health science curricula for training of health professionals in all disciplines (De Vries, Kathard and Müller 2020). The Psychological Society of South Africa has developed guidelines for psychology professionals working with sexually and gender diverse people (McLachlan et al. 2019). Trans people were involved in the core team who developed the guidelines. These guidelines can be used for mental health advocacy (Pillay et al. 2019). Widespread training on the guidelines has taken place and is ongoing. The guidelines are based on 12 statements that focus on equipping professionals with ethical, sensitive and affirming ways when engaging with sexually and gender diverse people (Victor, Nel, Lynch and Mbatha, 2014; PsySSA 2017). These guidelines also provide a framework for understanding the challenges that are created living in a patriarchal, hetero-cis-normative society and the impact that it has on gender diverse people (McLachlan et al. 2019).

New Models of Care

New models of care are evolving. The informed consent model, with a participatory approach, plays a vital role in the field of gender-affirming healthcare in South Africa (McLachlan 2019). The participatory approach endeavors to establish each TGD person as an agent of change within their community, as well as in public healthcare. The TGD individual does not only become the driver of their own medical transitioning, but also an ambassador for the trans and gender diverse community.

The participatory approach enables the TGD person to have autonomy in their transitioning. Through access to healthcare trainings and being empowered with knowledge and skills, the TGD person is able to engage within the community, not only about their own needs, but also establishing safe spaces for the TGD person. Gender affirming healthcare workers support the TGD person in their transitioning and they are seen as equal partners in the gender-affirming healthcare space. This approach not only enables the TGD person to be heard, but also to actively engage with the process of healthcare reform.

Conclusion

For many years the landscape has looked very bleak for TGD people in South Africa. Today, there are signs of hope, oases of possibility for improved access to care. Most encouragingly, trans people and organizations are playing an active role in educating trans communities and healthcare workers, and in developing guidelines for the delivery of gender-affirming care. The authors are hopeful that access to care will continue to improve in years to come.

References

De Vries, E.; Kathard, H. and Müller, A. (2020): Debate: Why should gender-affirming health care be included in health science curricula? In: BMC Medical Education, 20(1), 51.

Gabriel, N. (Ed.) (2016): Progressive Prudes – A survey of attitudes towards homosexuality & gender non-conformity in South Africa. Johannesburg: The Other Foundation.

Hamblin, R. and Nduna, M. (2013): Alteration of Sex Description and Sex Status Act and access to services for transgender people in South Africa. In: New Voices in Psychology, 9(1&2), pp. 50–62.

Hatchard, J. (1994): The Constitution of the Republic of South Africa. In: Journal of African Law, 38(1), pp. 70-77.

Hendricks, M.L. and Testa, R.J. (2012): A conceptual framework for clinical work with transgender and gender nonconforming clients: An adaptation of the minority stress model. In: Professional Psychology: Research and Practice, 43(5), pp. 460–467.

Husakouskaya, N. (2013): Rethinking gender and human rights through transgender and intersex experiences in South Africa. In: Agenda, 27(4), pp. 10–24.

Jobson, G.; Tucker, A.; De Swardt, G.; Rebe, K.; Struthers, H.; McIntyre, J. and Peters, R. (2018): Gender identity and HIV risk among men who have sex with men in Cape Town, South Africa. In: AIDS Care – Psychological and Socio-Medical Aspects of AIDS/HIV, 30(11), pp. 1421–1425.

Klein, T. (2012): Who Decides Whose Gender? Medico-legal classifications of sex and gender and their impact on transgendered South Africans' family rights. In: Ethnoscripts, 14(2), pp. 12–34.

Koch, J.M.; McLachlan, C.; Victor, C. J.; Westcott, J. and Yager, C. (2019): The cost of being transgender: where socio-economic status, global health care systems, and gender identity intersect. In: Psychology & Sexuality, 11(1-2), pp. 103-119.

Luvuno, Z.P.; Ncama, B. and Mchunu, G. (2019): Transgender population's experiences with regard to accessing reproductive health care in Kwazulu-Natal, South Africa: A qualitative study. In: Afr J Prim Health Care Fam Med, 11(1), pp. e1-e9.

Mayosi, B.M.; Lawn, J.E.; Van Niekerk, A.; Bradshaw, D.; Abdool Karim, S.S. and Coovadia, H.M. (2012): Health in South Africa: Changes and challenges since 2009. In: The Lancet, 380(9858), pp. 2029–2043.

McLachlan, C. (2019): Que(e)ring trans and gender diversity. In: South African Journal of Psychology, 49(1), pp. 7-9.

McLachlan, C.; Nel, J.A.; Pillay, S.R. and Victor, C.J. (2019): The Psychological Society of South Africa's guidelines for psychology professionals working with sexually and gender-diverse people: towards inclusive and affirmative practice. In: South African Journal of Psychology, 49(3), pp. 314-324.

Meer, T. and Müller, A. (2017): "They treat us like we're not there": Queer bodies and the social production of healthcare spaces. In: Health & Place, 45(May), pp. 92–98.

Mudarikwa, M.; May, C. and Martens, C. (Eds.) (2017): In Pursuit of Equality in South Africa – The Experiences of the Legal Resources Centre [online]. Johannesburg: Legal Resources Centre. Available at: https://lrc.org.za/wp-content/uploads/pdf/2017%20In%20Pursuit%20of%20Equality%20in%20South%20Africa.pdf (Accessed 29 November 2021).

Müller, A. (2016): Health for All? Sexual Orientation, Gender Identity, and the Implementation of the Right to Access to Health Care in South Africa. In: Health & Human Rights: An International Journal, 18(2), pp. 195–208.

Müller, A. (2017): Scrambling for access: availability, accessibility, acceptability and quality of healthcare for lesbian, gay, bisexual and transgender people in South Africa. In: BMC International Health and Human Rights, 17(16), pp. 1–10.

Müller, A.; Daskilewicz, K. and the Southern and East African Research Collective on Health (2019): Are we doing alright? Realities of violence, mental health, and access to healthcare related to sexual orientation and gender identity and expression in South Africa: Research report based on a community-led study in nine countries. Amsterdam: COC Netherlands.

National Essential Medicines List Committee (NEMLC, 2019): Tertiary and Quaternary Level Essential Medicines List. Reviewed Items. January 2020. Republic of South Africa: Department of Health. Available at: http://www.kznhealth.gov.za/pharmacy/Tertiary-quaternary-level-essential-medicine-recommendations_January2020.pdf (Accessed 29 November 2021).

Newman-Valentine, D.D. and Duma, S.E. (2014): Transsexual women's journey towards a heteronormative health care system. In: African Journal for Physical, Health Education, Recreation and Dance, 2(Supplement 1), pp. 385–394.

Nkoana, T. and Nduna, M. (2012): Engaging primary health care providers in transgender community health care: Observations from the field. New Voices in Psychology, 8(2), pp. 120–129.

Pillay, S.R.; Nel, J.A.; McLachlan, C. and Victor, C.J. (2019): Queering the history of South African psychology: From apartheid to LGBTI+ affirmative practices. American Psychologist, 74(8), pp. 954–966.

Psychological Society of South Africa (PsySSA, 2017): Practice guidelines for psychology professionals working with sexually and gender-diverse people [online]. Available at: https://www.psyssa.com/wp-content/uploads/2018/04/PsySSA-Diversity-Competence-Practice-Guidelines-PRINT-singlesided.pdf (Accessed 29 November 2021).

Reisner, S.L.; Poteat, T.; Keatley, J.A.; Cabral, M.; Mothopeng, T.; Dunham, E.; Holland, C.E.; Max, R. and Baral, S.D. (2016): Global health burden and needs of transgender populations: a review. In: The Lancet, 388(10042), pp. 412–436.

Republic of South Africa (2000): Government Gazette. Promotion of Equality and Prevention of Unfair Discrimination Act, No. 4 [online]. Available at: https://www.gov.za/sites/default/files/gcis_document/201409/a4-001.pdf (Accessed 29 November 2021).

Republic of South Africa (2003): Government Gazette. Alteration of Sex Description and Sex Status Act, No. 49 [online]. Available at: https://www.gov.za/sites/default/files/gcis_document/201409/a49-03.pdf (Accessed 29 November 2021).

Richter, M.; Chersich, M.; Temmerman, M. and Luchters, S. (2013): Characteristics, sexual behaviour and risk factors of female, male and transgender sex workers in South Africa. In: South African Medical Journal, 103(4), pp. 246–251.

Samudzi, Z. and Mannell, J. (2016): Cisgender male and transgender female sex workers in South Africa: gender variant identities and narratives of exclusion. In: Culture, Health and Sexuality, 18(1), pp. 1–14.

Sanger, N. (2014): Young and Transgender: Understanding the Experiences of Young Transgender Persons in Educational Institutions and the Health Sector in South Africa. A Gender DynamiX Report. Cape Town: Gender DynamiX.

South African National Aids Council (SANAC, 2012): National Strategic Plan on HIV, STIs and TB 2012-2016 [online]. Available at: https://www.gov.za/sites/default/files/gcis_document/201409/national-strategic-plan-hiv-stis-and-tb0.pdf (Accessed 29 November 2021).

South African National Aids Council (SANAC, 2017): Let our actions count: South Africa's national strategic plan for HIV, TB and STIs 2017-2022 [online]. Available at: https://sanac.org.za/wp-content/uploads/2017/06/NSP _FullDocument_FINAL.pdf (Accessed 29 November 2021).

Spencer, S.; Meer, T. and Müller, A. (2017): "The care is the best you can give at the time": Health care professionals' experiences in providing gender affirming care in South Africa. In: PLoS ONE, 12(7), pp. 1–18.

Stevens, M. (2012): Transgender access to sexual health services in South Africa: Findings from a key informant survey. Cape Town: Gender DynamiX.

Victor, C.J.; Nel, J.A.; Lynch, I. and Mbatha, K. (2014): The Psychological Society of South Africa sexual and gender diversity position statement: contributing towards a just society. In: South African Journal of Psychology, 44(3), pp. 292-302.

Wilson, D.; Marais, A.; De Villiers, A.; Addinall, R. and Campbell, M.M. (2014): Transgender issues in South Africa, with particular reference to the Groote Schuur Hospital Transgender Unit. In: South African Medical Journal, 104(6), p. 449.

No Data, No Problem?
Trans People and Healthcare in German Prisons

trans*Ratgeber Kollektiv

There is a conspicuous lack of official research and statistics regarding the number and the experiences of trans people imprisoned in Germany, in comparison with other countries such as the U.S.A., Australia, Austria or Italy (see Davis 2016; Spade 2011; Valerio 2018; Brömdal 2018; Czermak 2013; Vianello 2018). This lack of data makes it impossible to deliver a statistical overview of the German situation. This article covers the situation of some trans prisoners in Germany, their experiences and demands, as well as explaining the work of the "trans* Ratgeber collective Berlin". Instead of data, this article relies on oral testimony from the real experts: trans people detained in German prisons and psychiatric facilities.

About trans* Ratgeber Kollektiv

Our work includes ongoing research into legal precedents, by which we aim to better inform incarcerated trans people of their rights. We work to connect trans people in prison with lawyers and/or LGBTQIA+ support groups. In the process of offering this support, we have learned much about the situation of trans, non-binary and gender non-conforming people in German prisons.

Trans*Ratgeber Kollektiv has published a brochure containing legal and medical information and practical tips. The first edition of *"Informationen für trans* Menschen in Haft und Freund_innen und Unterstützer_innen"* (Informations for trans people in prison and their friends and supporters) was printed in 2018 and has been distributed to incarcerated people, prison libraries, prisoner support groups, LBGTQIA+ organizations and NGOs working in prisons around Germany. The brochure is currently being translated into several languages[1].

We are aware that intersex people and people with variations of physical sex characteristics suffer specific discriminations and violence both inside and outside prison. While these experiences differ from those of trans people, there are also overlapping topics and experiences of discrimination, especially the issues of placement (in a 'men's' or 'women's' prison), problems in accessing support groups, and medical needs such as hormone therapy.

Regrettably, trans* Ratgeber currently solely focuses on the situation of imprisoned trans people. We are working to broaden our contacts and increase our knowledge so that we can meaningfully support incarcerated intersex people and the intersex community.

Different Types of Prisons in Germany

We aim to support trans people incarcerated in prison (Strafvollzug), pretrial detention (Untersuchungshaft), juvenile detention (Jugendstrafvollzug), preventive detention (Sicherungsverwahrung), psychiatric prisons (Maßregelvollzug/Forensik) and immigration detention (Abschiebehaft).

Trans People in Immigration Detention

According to German law, people incarcerated in German migration detention centres can only be offered emergency medical care. Even then, such care is often denied (Pelzer and Sextro 2013).

So far, we have not been able to find any detailed information about the situation of trans* people in migration detention in Germany. However, we have read that throughout Europe, LGBTQIA+ refugees who have been denied asylum are often detained in isolation for long periods. They experience an increased rate of—sometimes even life-threatening—physical and sexual violence. This violence is perpetrated both by staff and by other detainees (Fütty 2019:158; Jansen and Spijkerboer 2011:77-78). Although data is lacking, it ap-

---

1   The brochure "Informationen für trans* Menschen in Haft und Freund_innen und Unterstützer_innen" is available for free download from http://transundhaft.blogsport.de. Printed copies can be ordered via email at transratgeber@gmx.de or via mail to trans* Ratgeber Gruppe, Bioladen Feuerbohne, Weichselstrasse 52, 12045 Berlin, Germany.

pears that it is very difficult for people in migration detention to get gender-affirming healthcare of any kind.

The Situation in German Prisons

Outside of prisons, trans people in Germany report that pervasive anti-trans sentiment obstructs access even to basic health care, let alone gender-affirming treatments. Inside prisons, limited medical care and violent enforcement of gender norms compound the discrimination trans people already face.

The gender binary of 'man' and 'woman' is a key concept within German prison law[2]. The law requires that men and women be imprisoned in separate facilities. This results in trans and intersex people being detained in prisons which do not match their gender, breaching the human right to gender self-determination and gender expression.

Since 2018, Germany legally recognizes a third gender called "diverse" (see Bundesgesetzblatt 2018). However, there is currently no legal guideline in cases of arrest or detention of a gender diverse person.

In Germany racial profiling is a common practice. Police stop and search Black people, People of Color, Rom_nija and people who are perceived to be Muslims at much higher rates than white people (see KOP – Kampagne für Opfer rassistischer Polizeigewalt 2019).

In the USA it is widely acknowledged that racial profiling is but one facet of the racist colonial justice system. Both cis and trans Black people, People of Color and First Nations people experience increased police harassment, are arrested and detained at disproportionately high rates and are subject to high rates of racist police violence, including killings by police (see Fütty 2019; Spade 2011; Davis 1989). One recent campaign that has brought public attention to racist police violence in the USA is #BlackLivesMatter (see Black Lives Matter 2020). So far, we have not found any statistics relating to rates of racist police profiling and violence in Germany.

Institutional racism is not only found in the justice system, but also the healthcare system, housing, education, and the jobs market. Medical racism exists in many countries including Germany. The consequences are, for example, that Black people and People of Color often experience discrimination when trying to access healthcare. Existing racism in German society doesn't disappear within prison walls; rather, it is amplified. This means that Black

---

2   The so called "separation principal paragraph" (Trennungsgrundsatz Paragraph) in the "penitentiary laws" (Strafvollzugsgesetze).

people and People of Color within the prison are likely to experience more violence and have even less access to healthcare, compared with white people in prison. For Black trans people and trans People of Color in prison, the situation is even worse, due to the intersectional oppressions that they face.

Support Organizations for Incarcerated Trans People in Germany

Several organizations in Germany are working on healthcare issues within prisons, but their focus tends to be on drug use and/or the prevention of HIV and hepatitis.

We don't know of any German LGBTQIA+ organizations that are officially working within the prison system to support trans people. However, we have heard of organizations such as TransInterQueer e.V., LesMigras, GLADT and Queer Leben in Berlin, as well as the Trans*beratung in Düsseldorf, that are working to support individual trans people in prisons. We are also aware of several more clandestine, less formal activist groups working on this topic and supporting incarcerated trans people, for example by writing letters to them. Writing letters to prisoners can help to break the violent isolation that they often face. Furthermore, trans prisoners may face additional seclusion due to anti-trans hate from prison staff and other prisoners. In many cases trans prisoners are also physically isolated from other prisoners. Writing to trans prisoners is a simple act of solidarity that may help to break the lived isolation so that feelings of loneliness do not become overpowering. Writing can also provide important information and gives the detainees a chance for their voice to be heard outside the prison walls. We try to give trans prisoners support and to empower them to fight for their rights.

We believe that trans people's healthcare needs should be an integral part of any discussion about prisons and health. This is why we presented a session focusing on the needs of incarcerated trans people at the *10th European Conference on Health Promotion in Custody* in Bonn, Germany, in 2019. We made use of the opportunity offered to present our work supporting trans people in custody and their specific health needs. The response of the audience was positive. Several psychologists, healthcare workers and social workers approached us after the presentation, emphasizing that they find this an important topic. Our general impression was that there is a significant lack of information about trans issues in prison life (see Gesund in Haft 2019).

Experiences of Trans People in German Prisons

We are in contact with a number of trans people imprisoned in Germany, who have shared their experiences with us so that we can offer support and connect them with resources and other organizations. These people have asked us to preserve their anonymity, to avoid putting them in danger or causing them additional harassment. For this reason, no names, prison types, or medical information are mentioned in the following accounts.

In conversations with people who have been incarcerated, we heard of one individual who requested a transfer from a male prison to a female prison. This person was able to transfer, but only after a legal fight. There are no official statistics regarding the number of people who have asked for a transfer to a different prison, according to their gender (Berliner Abgeordnetenhaus 2016).

Based on the right to gender self-determination, and the virulent anti-trans violence in prisons, we argue that trans people must have the option to choose whether to be incarcerated in a male or female prison.

It has been shown that violence harms people's mental and physical health, and trans people are exposed abundantly to violence inside and outside of the prison system. This may include anti-trans physical, sexualized, psychological and/or medical violence. Inside prisons, violence may come from both staff and prisoners.

Solitary confinement causes significant mental harm and has been recognized by human rights experts as a form of torture. "For many prisoners, solitary confinement is a sentence worse than death." (Bowers et al. 2014:8). We have received reports from trans people isolated in prisons, supposedly for their protection, as well as the maintenance of 'safety and order' in the prison. Although there are differences between solitary confinement and partial separation from the general prison population, we believe both are harmful and believe that research into the effects of isolation on trans people is needed. German laws regulate access to medical care. However, these laws are vague, which means that every medical institution and/or doctor may interpret them differently.

Outside of prison, many trans people find it hard to access healthcare (Veale et al. and the Canadian Trans Youth Survey Research Group 2015). A trans person might see many different doctors before they find someone understanding and knowledgeable about trans health. People incarcerated in Germany do not have the option to choose between different doctors, and it is very difficult to see a specialist. Prison doctors are part of the prison system and therefore are anything but 'neutral'. As well as being subject to violence from prison guards and other prisoners, trans people in prison may also experience violence at the hands of prison medical staff. In some cases, medical staff in prisons may choose to provide gender-affirming medical care, but when this care is denied, it is very difficult to challenge this decision. In theory, prisoners could take legal action to demand better healthcare, but as the laws applying to these cases are vague, this may require far greater time and legal resources than are available.

Trans people in German prisons report that, due to these structural barriers, it is extremely difficult for them to access gender-affirming medical care. Trans healthcare does not only include hormone therapy or gender reassignment surgery, it may also involve psychological support, regular endocrinological exams, lab tests, logopedic voice training, laser epilation, etc. Staff in German prisons lack general knowledge about trans related matters and are not equipped to provide adequate health care and general support for trans prisoners. We have received accounts from trans people imprisoned in Germany that transphobic stereotypes have been used as pretexts to deny them medical care. One person told us that he was denied gender-affirming testosterone therapy based on the misconception that 'higher testosterone levels would make him aggressive'. Incarcerated trans people have also reported that they were denied gender-affirming healthcare on the grounds that their sentence was 'not very long'—so they could wait until after their release to start gender-affirming treatments.

According to German law, new prisoners are supposed to receive a medical check-up. During this procedure, their medical needs are discussed with a prison medic. People who were officially undergoing gender-affirming hormone therapy before being imprisoned cannot be legally denied hormones while they are incarcerated. 'Official' eligibility for gender-affirming hormone therapy requires that the prisoner provide documentation of an F64 Gender Identity Disorder diagnosis under the ICD10[3] (International Classification of Diseases) guidelines (WHO n.d. a).

---

3   The "Working Group on Sexual Disorders and Sexual Health" has developed a different classification for trans for the updated ICD11: it speaks of "gender incongruence" (WHO n.d. b) The ICD11 classifications was supposed to come into force in Germany in January 2022.

For this reason, if a person was undergoing hormone therapy without medical supervision before imprisonment, it will likely not be possible to continue the treatment. Approval for continuation of gender-affirming hormone therapy may be possible but depends on the decision of the prison doctor.

Official statistics regarding the number of gender-affirming surgeries undergone by prisoners in Germany do not exist, but according to the Berlin Senate (Senat Berlin 2016), some prisoners in Berlin have had gender-affirming surgery. Due to doctor-patient confidentiality, the doctors in question are not able to speak about the procedures. Our collective, through personal contacts, are aware that some prisoners have requested and been denied gender-affirming surgery. The reason given was that 'it would not be possible for them to complete the needed aftercare while in prison'. Another person also told us that she was denied gender-affirming surgery while in prison and was also denied a detention break to undergo the surgery outside the prison.

Some people in prison have access to group or individual therapy. As the available therapists are part of the prison system, it is difficult for prisoners to develop the necessary relationship of trust with them. We received reports of trans people who were able to see a psychologist in prison, but they were not allowed to see an expert on trans healthcare. We have also heard of cases where the medical staff in psychiatric prisons were drugging incarcerated people to the point that they could barely walk.

In 2011 a trans woman in Celle, Germany, was denied the right to wear female clothes in prison. Prison authorities argued that if she wore women's clothing, she might be attacked. She went to court to fight the arbitrary decision and won the case: She was allowed to wear women's clothes and use make-up while in prison (Oberlandesgericht Celle 2011). The option to wear gender-affirming clothes can have a huge effect on a trans person's mental health. "People with GNC [*gender non-conforming*, the authors] identities and expressions face significant discrimination and victimization that contribute to the development of poorer mental, physical, and behavioral health." (Eckstrand, Ng and Potter 2016:1108). Although the above-mentioned case in Celle provides a legal precedent, it is not always easy for imprisoned people to access gender-affirming clothing and accessories. Some trans prisoners who contacted us mentioned that it is difficult for them to access important auxiliaries such as binders, packers, or breast prosthetics.

Another significant problem is that prisoners in Germany are generally denied internet access, and prison shops provide a limited—and binary gendered—range of items, especially cosmetics and sanitary products. This makes it difficult for trans people in prison to access even basic gender-affirming items like make-up, or personal care and hygiene products (shampoo, shower gel, aftershave, razors, hair-removal products, body lotion, deodorant, etc.).

One person told us that he was able to contact a trans-self-help organization while in prison, but in general, we do not know much about the extent to which trans people in prison can access support groups. As mentioned above, there are no specifically trans-focused organizations that operate inside German prisons.

Research is Lacking, But Incarcerated Trans People Have Clear Demands

We have received several reports from individuals talking about their particular experiences, but due to a lack of official documentation, it is impossible to get an overview of the overall situation of trans prisoners in Germany. We do not even know how many trans people have been incarcerated in Germany, nor do we know anything about the reasons they have been sentenced and whether anti-trans discrimination was a factor in their criminalization and imprisonment. Almost nothing is known about their most violent experiences inside prison, and we don't know what experiences they had after being released. It is very clear that more data about trans prisoners are needed. We advocate for ethical, participatory research with a special focus on the needs of trans prisoners.

Radical changes are needed to improve the situation of trans people in prisons. For example, trans people need to be able to choose which prison they are detained in (male/female). They should have the option to wear gender-affirming clothing and have access to cosmetics and other personal care and hygiene products necessary for adequate gender expression. Furthermore, gender-affirming medical treatment (including hormone therapy and gender-affirming surgeries) should be made available, and trans people should be legally allowed to change their name and gender while in prison.

Many improvements could be made to reduce the repression and discrimination faced by trans people in German prisons. To ensure these changes truly meet the needs of incarcerated trans people, it is necessary to heed the demands of current and former trans prisoners.

Prison Is a Mirror of Society

Prisons harm people's health. General medical care is lacking in all prisons, and trans people suffer from this on top of a lack of gender-affirming care. As a collective, we fight for better healthcare not only for trans prisoners, but for all prisoners. Prison systems should not be viewed as isolated institutions. They are a part of the society as a whole and they will never be better than the society of which they form part. Although we work to support trans people inside the prison system, in the long-term we are committed to prison abolition. Prisons exacerbate societal harms instead of fixing them. We need to address the root causes of poverty, addiction, homelessness, and mental illness instead of criminalizing them. To call for reform of the prison system without its abolition addresses only the symptoms, not the cause.

Most prisons outside Europe were established during colonization (see Dikötter 2007). In colonized countries, prisons "were part of an intense policy of taming political, economic and cultural resistance to white domination." (Bernault 2007:65-66). There are examples of non-western societies where violent conflicts are confronted with tools of transformative justice. We are committed to creating an equitable society—one that favors transformative justice approaches in dealing with cases of interpersonal violence, rather than locking people away (see Davis 2016).[4] Work to eliminate poverty, racism, (cis-)sexism and incarceration is inextricably linked with the work of eradicating interpersonal harm. Aside from improving the situation of trans prisoners, we strive for community accountability, social justice, freedom of movement and inclusive gender politics.

---

4   See also "World without Prisons" : https://www.worldwithoutprisons.org (13.02.2021). Organizations working in support of incarcerated trans people: Abo comix (www.abo-comix.com); Bent Bars (www.bentbarsproject.org); Black and Pink (www.blackand-pink.org); Immigration Equality (www.immigrationequality.org); Let's Get Free (www.letsgetfree.info); Sylvia Rivera Law Project (www.srlp.org); TGI Justice (www.tgijp.org); Trans Prisoner Day of Action and Solidarity – (www.transprisoners.wordpress.com); Black Lives Matter (https://www.blacklivesmatter.com/six-years-s trong/)

References

Berliner Abgeordnetenhaus (2016): Drucksache 18/10001 – Schriftliche Anfrage – Gender Trouble im Berliner Strafvollzug [online]. Available at: https://www.linksfraktion.berlin/fileadmin/linksfraktion/ka/2016/S18 -10001.pdf (Accessed 3 February 2022).

Bernault, F. (2007): The Shadow of Rule: Colonial Power and Modern Punishment in Africa. In: Frank Dikötter (Ed.): Cultures of Confinement: A Global History of the Prison in Asia, Africa, the Middle-East and Latin America. London: Christopher Hurst, pp. 55-94.

Black Lives Matter (2020): Six Years Strong [online]. Available at: https://blacklivesmatter.com/six-years-strong/ (Accessed 3 February 2021).

Bowers, M.; Fernandez, P.; Shah, M. and Slager, K. (2014): Solitary Confinement as Torture. Report by the University of North Carolina School of Law Immigration/Human Rights Clinic [Online]. Available at: https://law.unc.edu/wp-content/uploads/2019/10/solitaryconfinementreport.pdf (Accessed 11 February 2021).

Brömdal, A.; Mullens, A.B.; Phillips, T.M. and Gow, J. (2018): Experiences of transgender prisoners and their knowledge, attitudes, and practices regarding sexual behaviors and HIV/STIs: A systematic review. In: International Journal of Transgenderism, 20(1), pp. 4-20.

Bundesgesetzblatt (2018): Gesetz zur Änderung der in das Geburtenregister einzutragenden Angaben. Teil 1, Nr. 48, Bonn: Bundesanzeigerverlag.

Crenshaw, K. (1989): Demarginalizing the Intersection of Race and Sex: A Black Feminist Critique of Antidiscrimination Doctrine, Feminist Theory and Antiracist Politics [online]. Available at: https://philpapers.org/archive/CREDTI.pdf (Accessed 8 October 2019).

Czermak, Y. (2013): Von Paradiesvögeln, verzauberten Männern und Frauen in Tüten. Transidentität im Österreichischen Straf- und Maßnahmenvollzug. Unpublished Manuspript (Project report). Wien.

Davis, A.Y. (2016): Freedom is a constant struggle. Chicago, Illinois: Haymarket Books.

Dikötter, F. (Ed.) (2007): Cultures of Confinement: A Global History of the Prison in Asia, Africa, the Middle-East and Latin America. London: Christopher Hurst.

Eckstrand, K.L.; Ng, H. and Potter, J. (2016): Affirmative and Responsible Health Care for People with Nonconforming Gender Identities and Expressions. In: AMA Journal of Ethics, 18(11), pp. 1107-1119.

Franzen, J. and Sauer, A. (2010): Benachteiligung von Trans*Personen, insbesondere im Arbeitsleben. Expertise im Auftrag der Antidiskriminierungsstelle des Bundes [online]. Available at: https://www.antidiskri minierungsstelle.de/SharedDocs/downloads/DE/publikationen/Expertis en/expertise_benachteiligung_von_trans_personen.pdf?__blob=publicati onFile&v=3 (Accessed 03 February 2022).

Fütty, T.J.J. (2019): Gender und Biopolitik. Normative und intersektionale Gewalt gegen Trans*Menschen. Bielefeld: transcript.

Gesund in Haft (2019): Programm [online]. Available at: https://gesundinhaf t.eu/wp-content/uploads/ProgrammBonn19final.pdf (Accessed 8 October 2019).

KOP- Kampagne für Opfer rassistischer Polizeigewalt [online]. Available at: h ttps://kop-berlin.de/ueber-kop (Accessed 27 September 2019).

Kenagy, G.P. (2005): Transgender Health: Findings from Two Needs Assessment Studies in Philadelphia. In: Health & Social Work, 30(1), pp. 19–26.

Oberlandesgericht Celle (2011): Beschluss vom 9. Februar 2011, Az. 1, Ws 29/11 (StrVollz) [online]. Available at: https://openjur.de/u/326524.html (Accessed 26 September 2019).

Pelzer, M. and Sextro, U. (2013): Schutzlos hinter Gittern [online]. Available at: https://www.proasyl.de/wp-content/uploads/2015/12/PRO_ASYL_Beri cht_Abschiebungshaft_Juli_2013-1.pdf (Accessed 8 October 2019).

Senat Berlin (2015): Antwort auf die Schriftliche Anfrage Nr. 17/16621 vom 8. Juli 2015 über Gender Trouble im Berliner Strafvollzug [online]. Available at: https://www.berlin.de/justizvollzug/_assets/schriftliche-anfragen/s18 _10001_-_gender_trouble_im_berliner_strafvollzug.pdf (Accessed 08 August 2019).

Senat Berlin (2016): Schriftliche Anfrage des Abgeordneten Carsten Schatz (LINKE) vom 31. Oktober 2016 (Eingang beim Abgeordnetenhaus am 01. November 2016) und Antwort. Gender Trouble im Berliner Strafvollzug? Available at: https://www.linksfraktion.berlin/fileadmin/linksfraktion/ka /2016/S18-10001.pdf (Accessed 8 August 2019).

Spade, D. (2011): Normal Life. Brooklyn, NY: South End Press.

Spijkerboer, T. and Jansen, S. (2011): Fleeing Homophobia: Asylum Claims Related to Sexual Orientation and Gender Identity in the EU (September 6, 2011). Fleeing Homophobia: Asylum Claims Related to Sexual Orientation and Gender Identity in the EU [online]. Available at: https://ssrn.com/ab stract=2097783 (Accessed 10 October 2019).

TSG (1980): Gesetz über die Änderung der Vornamen und die Feststellung der Geschlechtszugehörigkeit in besonderen Fällen [online]. Available at: h ttps://www.gesetze-im-internet.de/tsg/BJNR016540980.html (Accessed 1 August 2019).

Valerio, P.; Bertolazzi, C.; Marcasciano, P.; Hochdorn, A. and Sicca, L.M. (2018): Transformare l'organizzazione dei luoghi di detenzione. Persone transgender e gender nonconforming tra diritti e identità. Napoli: Editoriale Scientifica.

Veale, J.; Saewyc, E.M.; Frohard-Dourlent, H.; Dobson S.; Clark, B. and Canadian Trans Youth Survey Research Group (2015): Being Safe, Being Me: Results of the Canadian Trans Youth Health Survey. Vancouver, BC: Stigma and Resilience Among Vulnerable Youth Centre, School of Nursing, University of British Columbia.

Vianello, F.; Vitelli, R.; Hochdorn, A. and Mantovan, C. (2018): Che genere di carcere? Il sistema penitenziario alla prova delle detenute transgender. Milano: Guerini e Associati.

World Health Organization (n.d. a): ICD-10 – Version 2016. F64.0 Transsexualism [online]. Available at: https://icd.who.int/browse10/2016/en#/F64.0 (Accessed 3 February 2022).

World Health Organization (n.d. b): International Classification of Diseases 11th Revision – The global standard for diagnostic health information [online]. Available at: https://icd.who.int/en (Accessed 3 February 2022).

Community-Driven Responses to Public Health: An Example from England's HIV Sector

Aedan Wolton and Matthew Hibbert

> "We call on researchers to include transgen-
> der women, men, and non-binary people,
> who are at risk of or living with HIV in their
> research.
> [...] Sitting in the audience or appearing
> in photos in a slide deck does not con-
> stitute meaningful involvement of trans
> colleagues."
> *(Scheim et al. 2019)*

Trans Healthcare in England and the UK

Recent years have seen a significant rise in the number of trans/non-binary adults seeking to undergo some form of medically supervised transition via the National Health Service (NHS) in England (The Tavistock and Portman NHS Foundation Trust 2019); with an estimated 240% increase in referrals to England's seven publicly funded Gender Identity Clinics (GICs) between 2013 and 2018 (Torjesen 2018). However, patient numbers from NHS GICs are generally considered to be a poor measure of the overall size of England's trans population. These figures fail to account for the many trans/non-binary people who have already been discharged from NHS services, as well as those who are sourcing gender affirming services abroad (or via private clinics in the UK), and those who acquire hormone therapy without medical supervision. Additionally, GIC patient numbers cannot take into account the number of trans/non-binary people who do not desire (or are unable to seek) medical interventions (Wolton et al. 2018).

These factors combined with the current lack of trans-inclusive national census data (and the fact that the wider NHS only records binary gender markers) mean that the total number of trans people living in England and throughout the rest of the UK is currently unknown. However, the UK is considered likely to be comparable to the US and other high-income countries, suggesting that 0.6% of the population may be gender diverse (Flores et al. 2016).

Without meaningful knowledge of the overall population size, generating accurate prevalence data for a number of health conditions in the UK's trans populations remains an impossibility. This, in turn, impacts the ways in which funding streams for both research and frontline services are allocated and contributes to the numerous ways in which trans/non-binary people are left behind by English healthcare provision.

In addition to the lack of inclusion in data monitoring across our healthcare systems, trans people also face a number of barriers when attempting to access services provided by the NHS, despite its constitutional commitment to timely, respectful, patient-centered healthcare for all (Department of Health and Social Care 2012). Waiting times for gender-affirming interventions in England are currently in excess of two years from point of referral to first appointment (Devon Partnership NHS Trust 2019). This is despite clear stipulation that no NHS patients (irrespective of gender identity) should wait longer than 18 weeks from the point of referral to the person's first specialist, consultant-led appointment (Department of Health and Social Care 2012).

For those in England who have had no viable alternative but to wait for publicly funded care, the barriers to gender affirmation extend way beyond the time it takes to be assessed by an NHS gender identity service. These specialist, multidisciplinary clinics do not provide hormone therapy directly. Instead, GICs assess and diagnose Gender Dysphoria (American Psychiatric Association 2013) and subsequently make recommendations for the individual's general practitioner (GP) to commence hormone therapy under their supervision.

Whilst this offers a theoretically acceptable model of shared care delivery, this is often not the reality in practice. As many as one-in-five NHS GPs will go on to refuse to prescribe hormones to their trans/non-binary patients (Barrett, 2016). With these pitfalls well known at the community level, it is unsurprising that as many as 40% of trans/non-binary people will be self-sourcing hormone therapy (without medical supervision) by the time they attend their first NHS GIC appointment (Mepham et al. 2014).

Years of vocal community activism have brought political focus to the numerous issues trans people experience both in and beyond the UK's healthcare systems. As a result, in 2016, the UK Government's Women and Equalities Committee undertook a national inquiry into trans equality. The subsequent report concluded that the NHS is largely failing trans/non-binary people. It described the standard of care delivered by various sections of the health service as discriminatory and often in breach of England's national equality legislation (Women and Equalities Committee 2016). A later government survey also found that nearly half of trans/non-binary people in the UK had reported at least one negative experience of NHS services in 2017-2018 (Government Equalities Office 2018). Long waiting times appear as a significant contributor to these negative experiences:

> The waiting lists for GICs need genuine change [...] I have personally used alcohol, cannabis, cocaine and self-harm to survive the last year and a half since referral, and I have now been told I will have to wait several more months because of the backlog. (Trans man, heterosexual, 18-24, North West) (ibid.)

These difficulties are not unique to the UK. In many ways, the health of UK trans populations is comparable to those of other nations across the globe. Self-harm and suicidality are common. Trans/non-binary people throughout the UK often have poor mental and physical health outcomes (McNeil et al. 2012), and in some metropolitan areas, also experience complications relating to the late diagnosis of HIV (Suchak et al. 2017).

Additionally, the high incidence of unsupervised hormone usage (Mepham et al. 2014) coupled with increased rates of problematic drinking, smoking and substance use within the community (McNeil et al. 2012) pose a significant and under-researched risk of adverse cardiovascular events within this population. Pockets of existing knowledge are generally derived from local or small-scale studies, as erasure of trans populations has, historically, extended to a lack of inclusion in national public health research either as participants or as researchers. This lack of trans/non-binary visibility causes particular difficulties in relation to HIV, since accurate monitoring of the epidemic's progression is essential for understanding health needs, determining public health priorities, allocating resources, and evaluating the efficacy of interventions (Nsbuga et al. 2006).

Trans-led Inclusion in the UK's HIV Research

Approximately 32 million people across the globe have died from complications related to HIV since the early years of the epidemic (WHO 2019). Whilst significant breakthroughs in both preventing and treating the virus have been made in recent years, HIV transmission persists as a major public health concern and affects more than two million people in the World Health Organization (WHO) European Region. Whilst epidemic patterns vary by country, nearly 160,000 people across the region were diagnosed with HIV in 2017 (ECDC 2018).

The WHO, in a bid to reduce onward transmission, has called for international prevention efforts to focus on communities that are most vulnerable to acquiring the virus: substance users, men who have sex with men, sex workers, prisoners, and trans people. These 'key populations' are most at risk of becoming HIV positive and face significantly higher rates of HIV than the general population, accounting for more than 50% of new diagnoses (UNAIDS 2019).

Whilst meaningful HIV prevalence data relating to trans populations remain scarce, meta-analysis of existing studies suggests that as many as 19.1% of transgender women could be living with HIV across the globe (Baral, et al. 2013). Despite these alarming figures, 61% of UN countries, as recently as 2014, failed to include trans/non-binary people in their national HIV strategies or in their national epidemiological reporting (UNAIDS 2014). This, until recently, was also the case in England.

The earliest known efforts to collect meaningful, trans-inclusive sexual health and HIV data within an NHS context, emerged at a local level in 2013. 56 Dean Street, a leading sexual health & HIV clinic in Central London, began piloting an adapted version of Sausa et al.'s (2009) two-stage method of gender identity monitoring in their specialist trans/non-binary sexual health clinic. The service, which is a partnership between trans/non-binary professionals and a number of cisgender colleagues, uses registration forms that collect data concerning service users' current gender identity, as well as their sex assigned at birth.

Following the success of the Sausa et. al. (2009) model at Dean Street, it was adapted and refined for nationwide usage. This involved collaboration between a group of trans/non-binary professionals, Public Health England (PHE), the government agency responsible for England's national HIV reporting, and a number of key trans and LBGTQ-led organizations. The model was subsequently included in the People Living with HIV (PLWHIV) Stigma Index in 2015. The latter became the first government-sponsored national research initiative to include trans/non-binary populations in HIV survey data. It recruited participants over the age of 18 who were living with HIV from over 120 different community organizations and 46 NHS clinics across the UK.

The survey explored how and in what circumstances and locations (e.g., family events, religious contexts, healthcare settings etc.) participants either experienced or anticipated HIV-related stigma and how this intersected with other commonly stigmatized factors such as age, ethnicity, disability or trans status. Among the 1576 participants, 31 (2%) identified as trans in some way. It was found that trans people living with HIV were more likely than their cisgender counterparts to report negative experience of health services. They were also more likely to report feeling that they had received intentionally delayed treatment or that their treatment had been refused when attempting to access healthcare services in a range of settings (Hibbert et al. 2018).

Additionally, trans respondents exhibited greater psychosocial complexity in comparison to cis respondents, including higher rates of injection drug use, and a greater likelihood of having engaged in transactional sex. Whilst only a small proportion of participants identified as trans, this study highlighted the differences in the care that trans PLWHIV in the UK may receive. However, it is not possible to ascertain how representational this data is in relation to the experiences of all trans PLWHIV, as the prevalence of HIV was still unknown at the time of the study (ibid.).

Despite the small number of trans/non-binary respondents, The Stigma Index UK study marked an important turning point in the inclusion of trans people as expert researchers within the UK's HIV sector. It was a community-led project and was collaboratively created with an advisory group which included trans/non-binary people and other key populations vulnerable to or living with HIV. The study's collection of meaningful gender identity data, alongside effective trans-led community advocacy, became the catalyst for Public Health England to continue to include gender diverse populations in its national HIV surveillance. This included updates to its HIV/AIDS Reporting System (HARS); a public health coding and reporting tool which is utilized in all English and Welsh HIV services to effectively monitor the spread of HIV. Alongside this emerging clinical data, in 2017 PHE also went on to capture the lived experiences of trans/non-binary people in its Positive Voices Survey (an exploration of the lives, experiences and healthcare needs of PLWHIV in the UK) with responses to the survey validated using data triangulation and clinical follow-up.

PHE found that 0.19% (178/94,885) of people accessing HIV care in England and Wales in 2017 identified as trans/non-binary in some way. Of these, 140 (79%) identified as women, 12 (7%) as men, 20 (11%) as non-binary and 6 (3%) described their gender in another way. Unlike a number of other nations who have included trans/non-binary populations in HIV surveillance, rates of late diagnosis, antiretroviral uptake, and viral suppression were similar amongst trans and cis people (Kirwan et al. 2021).

PHE also found that trans PLWHIV were significantly more likely to be London residents (57% vs 43%) and were younger than their cisgender counterparts. Significantly, trans respondents were more likely than cis individuals to be under active psychiatric care (11% vs. 4%), were more likely to self-report anxiety and depression (41% vs. 24%) and, as previously found in the Stigma Index UK in 2015, were more likely to have been refused or delayed treatment in various healthcare settings. The Positive Voices Survey also highlighted that trans/non-binary people were more likely to describe their health as bad or very bad, as well as more likely to report problems with activities of daily living such as washing and dressing (ibid.).

In stark contrast to a number of non-UK studies, PHE found that trans/non-binary PLWHIV were more likely to be from white backgrounds, whereas the burden of HIV in trans people globally is predominantly experienced by trans women of color (Baral et al. 2013). This unexpected finding may be the result of the ways in which the dominant culture in the UK erases and excludes those from Latin American backgrounds from identifying as people of color; as a result, the NHS data dictionary does not allow health services to explicitly record Latin American ethnicities (NHS 2020). Instead, data is likely collected under the vague and erroneous heading of 'Any other white background'. However, Latin American people in the UK have been identified as a key population for HIV prevention (Rawson et al., 2019), and therefore understanding the number (and needs) of trans people of color, including Latin American trans people, in relation to HIV is essential for providing an optimum level of care in the UK in future.

UK Epidemiology and Implications for Further Research

Despite drawing attention to a number of disparities in the context of mental health and broader wellbeing, these early data from PHE suggest that HIV rates in trans people living in England may be significantly lower than a number of countries which have contributed to global prevalence estimates of 19.1% (Baral et al. 2013). However, the mechanism for capturing diverse gender identity data remains new and unfamiliar to predominantly cisgender clinicians, thus highlighting a significant need for the upscaling of training provisions. Until usage is improved, it can be assumed that inaccurate reporting or underreporting will occur. Additionally, the lack of a national trans/non-binary population figure dictates that prevalence data derived from the report can only be estimated at this time.

Significantly, despite its numerous difficulties in sensitively responding to the needs of trans/non-binary populations, England's free-at-the-point-of-access healthcare may be a contributing factor to the lower-than-expected estimate of HIV in trans people in comparison to the global figures. However, trans/non-binary people may be significantly underrepresented in the numbers of people accessing HIV care, as they are understood to be less likely to access sexual health services than their cisgender counterparts (Government Equalities Office 2018; Hibbert et al. 2020). In addition, when trans people do access sexual healthcare, they are more likely than cisgender people to rate the experience as negative (Government Equalities Office 2018) which could result in individuals not returning for necessary follow-up treatment and care.

The likelihood of losing trans/non-binary patients to follow-up could be reduced by restructuring our HIV services to be more responsive to the needs of our gender diverse communities. Currently, the UK health system is siloed by health condition or medical specialty, such that gender affirming services operate separately from sexual health and HIV care. However, existing research suggests that TPLWHIV consider hormone therapy to be a greater priority to their health than their HIV treatment (Schneiders 2014). Thus, the co-delivery of gender affirming interventions within existing sexual health and HIV services has the potential to increase long-term retention in care. London's 56 Dean Street will in 2020 become the first service in the UK to pilot a multidisciplinary model of this kind.

Despite these advances in service delivery, further academic attention is needed to assess the prevalence of undiagnosed HIV in trans/non-binary people in the UK. Additionally, further research is needed to understand how to increase the uptake of HIV testing within trans communities, as current reports are conflicting. One UK-wide study observed that trans people who exhibit HIV 'risk behaviors' are more likely to attend sexual health services (compared to trans people who experience less risk) and that they were more likely to have an HIV test (Hibbert et al. 2020).

However, pockets of risk have been identified in a small-scale, locality-specific study of trans/non-binary people who accessed a community-led outreach project at a sex-on-premises venue in London. The study found that over half of trans service users had engaged in condomless anal sex in the previous 6 months. However, just over a quarter of the 133 participants reported having tested for HIV in the last year, and the vast majority had no pre-existing knowledge of biomedical HIV prevention methods (i.e., pre- or post-exposure prophylaxis) (Wolton et al., 2018). Comparably, Hibbert et al. (2020) identified that half of trans people who reported condomless anal sex in the preceding 12 months had not attended a sexual health clinic that year.

Whilst both studies took into account various intersections of HIV vulnerability that trans/non-binary people may experience (substance use, sex work status etc.), neither explored the migration status of its participants (as was also the case in the Stigma Index and Positive Voices Surveys). Studies undertaken in non-UK countries demonstrate that undocumented migration status is emerging as a high-risk factor for HIV vulnerability amongst trans/non-binary populations (Palazzolo et al. 2016). Therefore, future UK studies should pay greater attention to migration status.

Conclusion: The Impact of Meaningful Inclusion on Clinical Practice

Whilst there are still a number of areas that require further, more detailed exploration, it is thanks to effective and consistent trans/non-binary community advocacy in the UK's HIV sector that gender diverse populations are able to be counted for the first time. Additionally, partnership between trans and LGBT+ organizations, trans/non-binary professionals, and the British Association of Sexual Health & HIV (BASHH) has led to the publication of comprehensive recommendations for *Integrated Sexual Health Services for Trans, Including Non-binary, People*. This document provides the first detailed recommendations (both clinical and non-clinical) on best practice when delivering sexual health services that are inclusive to gender diverse communities (BASHH 2019).

Sexual health and HIV research is becoming more inclusive for trans people as participants, researchers and collaborators. This sharing of knowledge and experiences has led to some significant changes in UK research and has also driven change at a frontline level. Effective trans leadership and inclusion has led to the commissioning of a new specialist sexual health and HIV service for trans/non-binary people in South London, the launch of TransPlus, the aforementioned pilot of a sexual health-based gender affirmation clinic. It has also fostered improved trans inclusion in existing sexual health initiatives, including the UK's National HIV Testing Week and a 56 Dean Street's PRIME service, a digital, smart phone intervention for men who have sex with men (MSM) that experience an increased likelihood of acquiring HIV (Nwokolo et al. 2017).

It is hard to imagine that the above would have been possible without consistent, effective advocacy from trans/non-binary communities both as leaders and patient advocates. Too often trans people are constructed as passive recipients of health services, rather than those who drive strategic innovation and positive change in the delivery of health services. It is only inclusion of and leadership from trans/non-binary people in the design and delivery of research, services and policy initiatives that has improved sexual health services in the UK for trans/non-binary communities. It is trans people who fought for their voices to be represented in amongst the narratives of those living with HIV in the UK. From that small spark, we believe there is a fire of radical, meaningful inclusion that is spreading throughout health systems in the UK at both national and local levels.

References

American Psychiatric Association (2013): Diagnostic and statistical manual of mental disorders (5th ed.). Washington DC: American Psychiatric Association.

Barratt, J. (2016): Doctors Are Failing to Help People with Gender Dysphoria. In: British Medical Journal, 352, p. i1694.

Baral, S.; Poteat, T.; Stromdahl, S.; Wirtz, A.; Guadamuz, T. and Beyrer, C. (2013): Worldwide Burden of HIV in Transgender Women: A Systematic Review and Meta-analysis. In: The Lancet Infectious Diseases, 13(3), pp. 214–222.

British Association of Sexual Health and HIV (BASHH, 2019): BASHH Recommendations For Integrated Sexual Health Services For Trans, Including

Non-Binary, People [online]. Available at: https://www.bashh.org/about-bashh/publications/ (Accessed: 02 December 2021).

Department of Health and Social Care (2012): The NHS Constitution for England [online]. Available at: https://www.gov.uk/government/publicat ions/the-nhs-constitution-for-england/the-nhs-constitution-for-englan d (Accessed: 02 December 2021).

Devon Partnership NHS Trust (2019): Accessing Our Services [online]. Available at: https://www.dpt.nhs.uk/our-services/gender-identity/for-people -using-our-service/accessing-our-service (Accessed: 02 December 2021).

European Centre for Disease Prevention and Control (ECDC, 2018): WHO Regional Office for Europe. HIV/AIDS Surveillance in Europe 2018 – 2017 data. Copenhagen: WHO Regional Office for Europe.

Flores, A.; Herman, J.; Gates, G. and Brown, T.N.T. (2016): How Many Adults Identify as Transgender in The United States? [online]. Los Angeles, CA: The Williams Institute. Available at: https://williamsinstitute.law.ucla.ed u/wp-content/uploads/Trans-Adults-US-Aug-2016.pdf (Accessed: 02 December 2021).

Government Equalities Office (2018): National LGBT Survey. Research Report [online]. Available at: https://assets.publishing.service.gov.uk/governme nt/uploads/system/uploads/attachment_data/file/721704/LGBT-survey-r esearch-report.pdf (Accessed: 02 December 2021).

Hibbert, M.; Wolton, A.; Crenna-Jennings, W.; Benton, L.; Kirwan, P.; Lut, I.; Okala, S.; Ross, M.; Furegato, M.; Nambiar, K.; Douglas, N.; Roche, J.; Jeffries, J.; Reeves, I.; Nelson, M.; Weerawardhana, C.; Zahra, J.; Hudson, A. and Delpech, V. (2018): Experiences of Stigma and Discrimination in Social and Healthcare Settings Among Trans People Living with HIV in the UK. In: AIDS Care, 30(9), pp. 1189-1196.

Hibbert, M.; Wolton, A.; Weeks, H.; Ross, M., Brett, C.E.; Porcellato, L.A. and Hope, V.D. (2020): Psychosocial and Sexual Factors Associated with Recent Sexual Health Clinic Attendance and HIV Testing Among Trans People in the UK. In: British Medical Journal, Sexual & Reproductive Health, 46(2), pp. 116-125.

Joint United Nations Programme on HIV/AIDS (UNAIDS, 2014): Global AIDS Response and Progress Reporting 2014 [online]. Available at: https://ww w.unaids.org/sites/default/files/media_asset/GARPR_2014_guidelines_e n_0.pdf (Accessed: 02 December 2021).

Joint United Nations Programme on HIV/AIDS (UNAIDS, 2019): Fact sheet-World Aids Day 2021 [online]. Available at: https://www.unaids.org/site

s/default/files/media_asset/UNAIDS_FactSheet_en.pdf (Accessed 02 December 2021).

Kirwan, P.; Hibbert, M.; Kall, M.; Nabiar, K.; Ross, M.; Webb, L.; Wolton, A. and Delpech, V. (2021): HIV prevalence and clinical outcomes of trans people living with HIV in England. In: HIV Medicine, 22(2), pp. 131-139.

McNeil, J.; Bailey, L.; Ellis, S.; Morton, J. and Regan, M. (2012): Trans mental health and emotional wellbeing study [online]. Available at: https://www.gires.org.uk/assets/Medpro-Assets/trans_mh_study.pdf (Accessed: 02 December 2021).

Mepham, N.; Bouman, W.; Arcelus, J.; Hayter, M. and Wylie, K. (2014): People with Gender Dysphoria Who Self-Prescribe Cross-sex Hormones: Prevalence, Sources, and Side Effects Knowledge. In: Journal of Sexual Medicine, 11(12), pp. 2995–3001.

National Health Service (NHS, 2020): NHS Data Model and Dictionary: Ethnic Category [online]. Available at: https://datadictionary.nhs.uk/data_elements/ethnic_category.html (Accessed: 02 December 2021).

Nsubuga, P.; White, M.; Thacker, S.; Anderson, M.; Blount, S.; Broome, C.; Chiller, T.; Espitia, V.; Imtiaz, R.; Sosin, D.; Stroup, D.; Tauxe, R.V.; Vijayaraghavan, M. and Trostle, M. (2006): Public Health Surveillance: A Tool for Targeting and Monitoring Interventions. In: Jamison, D.T.; Breman, J.G.; Measham, A.R.; Alleyne, G.; Claeson, M.; Evans, D.B.; Jha, P.; Mills, A. and Musgrove, P. (Eds.): Disease Control Priorities in Developing Countries (2nd edition). Washington, DC: The International Bank for Reconstruction and Development, Chapter 53.

Nwokolo, N.; Hill, A.; McOwan, A. and Pozniak, A. (2017): Rapidly Declining HIV Infections in MSM in Central London. In: The Lancet HIV, 4(11), pp. e482-e483.

Palazzolo, S.; Yamanis, T.; De Jesus, M. ; Maguire-Marshall, M. ; and Barker, S. (2016): Documentation Status as a Contextual Determinant of HIV Risk Among Young Transgender Latinas. In: LGBT Health, 3(2), pp. 132-138.

Rawson, S.; Croxford, S.; Swift, B.; Kirwan, P., Guerra, L. and Delpech, V. (2019): Latin Americans in the UK: A Key Population for HIV Prevention. In: HIV Medicine, 20(5), p. 54.

Sausa, L.; Sevelius, J.; Keatley, J.; Rouse Iñiguez, J. and Reyes, M. (2009): Policy Recommendations for Inclusive Data Collection of Trans People in HIV Prevention, Care & Services [online]. Available at: https://prevention.ucsf.edu/transhealth/education/data-recs-long (Accessed: 02 December 2021).

Scheim, A.; Appenroth, M.; Beckham, S.W.; Goldstein, Z.; Cabral Grinspan, M.; Keatley, J. and Radix, A. (2019): Transgender HIV Research: Nothing About Us Without Us. In: The Lancet HIV, 6(9), pp. 566-567.

Schnieders, M. (2014): Values and Preferences of Transgender People: A Qualitative Study [online]. Available at: http://apps.who.int/iris/bitstream/1 0665/128119/1/WHO_HIV_2014.21_eng.pdf?ua=1 (Accessed: 02 December 2021).

Suchak, T.; Patel, S.; Byrne, R.; Ross, M. and Wolton, A. (2017): Highly Invisible, Highly Infectious and High risk: The Hidden Problem of Trans People Living with HIV. 23rd Annual Conference of the British HIV Association (BHIVA), 04-07 April 2017.

The Tavistock and Portman NHS Foundation Trust (2019): Gender Identity Clinic: Waiting Times [online]. Available at: https://gic.nhs.uk/appointm ents/waiting-times/ (Accessed: 02 December 2021).

Torjesen, I. (2018): Trans Health Needs More and Better Services: Increasing Capacity, Expertise, and Integration. In: The British Medical Journal, 362, p. k3371.

Wolton, A.; Cameron, R.; Ross, M. and Suchak, T. (2018): Trans: Mission – A community-led HIV testing initiative for trans people and their partners at a Central London sex-on-premises venue. In: HIV Nursing Issue, 18(2/2018), pp. 24-29.

Women and Equalities Committee (2016): Transgender Equality. First report of Session 2015-16 [online]. London: House of Commons. Available at: https://publications.parliament.uk/pa/cm201516/cmselect/cmwomeq/ 390/390.pdf (Accessed: 02 December 2021).

World Health Organization (WHO, 2019): The Global Health Observatory Data. Explore a world of health data: HIV/AIDS [online]. Availble at: ht tps://www.who.int/data/gho/data/themes/hiv-aids (Accessed: 02 December 2021).

Cultural Competency with Non-Binary and Genderqueer Individuals: Results from a Qualitative Participatory Action Research Pilot Study

Sasha D. Strong, Sagan Wallace, Caleb Feldman & J. Ruby Welch

How can counselors and other health professionals acknowledge, include, and support non-binary (NB), genderqueer (GQ), and other gender non-conforming people? This study grew from the needs of a peer support group for non-binary and genderqueer people in Portland, Oregon, USA, and our wish to share our insights with the world. Based on our personal experiences of erasure, marginalization, invisibility, and being misunderstood and trivialized within mainstream cisheteropatriarchal culture and within the LGBTQ and trans communities, we want to make concrete recommendations for improving services for people like us[1]. This article blends an activist approach with a social science research project, with the hope that we will be able to leverage some of the power of scientific discourse in order to make change. We have tried to write for lay and professional audiences, and we hope that readers will bear with us as they navigate this hybrid text.

In the summer of 2017, we decided to conduct a participatory action research study using a qualitative thematic analysis method (Braun and Clarke

---

[1] (Sasha Strong) am the primary author of this research report, and I am the member of our group with the most formal training in qualitative research. In this report, I use 'we' when I am talking about what I sense is the collective voice of our research group based in our findings, and 'I' when I am speaking from my personal perspective as a researcher and clinician. Because our study is community-based, yet informed by scholarship and professional practice, in this report, I try to walk the line between scholarly language and plain speech, so that our findings can be easily put to use in counseling and healthcare by people from all walks of life.

2006). From our peer support group, we recruited seven non-binary and genderqueer people ($N = 7$, including the authors) and asked them their opinions on how to improve counselors' cultural competency. In this chapter, we start by defining and contextualizing non-binary and genderqueer issues, and we review some of the literature about folks like us. Next, we explain how we collected and analyzed the data for this research project. Then we present our findings in terms of 5 themes (Validation Basics, Holding Space for Complexity, Finding Safe Spaces, Erasure, and Trauma-Informed Intersectionality) and 12 best-practices. After that, we wrap up with a discussion of the implications of these findings and the limitations of this study.

In general, we hope that these findings will be applied to counseling, and generalized to healthcare and other human service fields, in order to improve relationships, communications, and gender assumptions with non-binary, genderqueer, and other gender-nonconforming people. Hopefully, this chapter will also help non-binary, genderqueer, and other gender diverse people understand their own position better, feel appreciated and understood, and help them to advocate for meaningful change in their lived contexts, in healthcare and beyond.

Even better, we hope this chapter will inspire gender diverse folks to engage in educational and research activism. This study is an example of participatory action research that can be replicated by other oppressed groups, and by non-binary, genderqueer, and other gender non-conforming people advocating for their needs in other contexts. Participatory action research has the potential to empower communities to work for recognition and systemic change, as well as to create communities of inquiry and practice. Dear reader: We appreciate you, and we hope you will join us in this work.

Definitions and Contextualization

The terms *genderqueer* and *non-binary* refer to aspects of gender identity, expression, and performance that go beyond the strict binary division of gender into only two categories of male and female. Whereas gender diversity and different forms of transness are gaining increasing recognition as a bona fide life experience, mainstream understanding, and portrayal of transgenderism is predominantly of binary gender changes, in which a person, who was assigned a male or female gender at birth goes through a process of self-discovery, social recognition, and medical transition to the opposite (binary) gender. While such binary trans experiences are valid and important, for us and people like us, it is clear that there are more than just two gender options. 'Non-binary' and 'genderqueer' are two words that some people (including the authors) choose to use to identify our lived experience, although some members of the group also sometimes use other words to describe themselves and their gender experience. (Isn't it wonderful how we're all different?)

A significant factor that shapes our lives is that our unique gender experience is routinely erased from public awareness, leading to significant social stress. For example, lavatories, clothing, medical forms, courtship customs, popular song, and most widely spoken languages and linguistic conventions constantly sort people into two (and only two) categories of male and female. For folks with a binary gender identity, there are specific life role experiences that mark and validate social identity, but non-binary and genderqueer folks do not have access to these same aspects of social approbation and understanding. Non-binary and genderqueer people can experience the same sorts of social stress and microaggression as binary trans- and cis-gender sexual minority individuals. To top it off, our experience is erased, ignored, and marginalized as we are repeatedly misgendered by strangers who automatically read us by appearance and performance, sort us into the male or female box, and blithely greet us as "sir" or "ma'am." In bathrooms, clothing stores, and health centers, we are repeatedly reminded of the gender binary and its assumption that people like us simply do not exist.

This is not to deny or ignore the other forms of pain and oppression that occur within cisheteropatriarchy, but simply to speak about our experience, as well. Clearly, cisgender women experience oppression in patriarchal culture, and cisgender men also experience constrained social roles and different kinds of marginalization. Binary trans men and trans women also experience identity-based oppression and marginalization, as attested by the epidemiological data (e.g., James et al. 2016). Non-binary, genderqueer, and other gender non-conforming people experience additional styles of social stigma, marginalization, denial of access to resources, microaggressions, and social violence due solely to our identity, experience, performance, and appearance in relation to our gender positionality. This chapter makes specific recommendations for how health professionals can provide a culturally competent experience for folks like us.

Non-Binary and Genderqueer Genders in the Literature

Non-binary, genderqueer, and other gender non-conforming experiences have received increasing attention in academic literature in the last several years, including the recent publication of an edited volume devoted to the topic (Richards, Bouman and Barker 2017). However, the topic was virtually invisible in the academic literature until recently: a 2016 PubMed[2] search for 'non-binary' and 'genderqueer' yielded a total of 59 results (54 and 5, respectively; Richards et al. 2016). At the time of writing in 2019, a similar search yields 222 results (171 for 'non-binary,' 51 for 'genderqueer'). Research into non-binary and genderqueer issues remains urgently needed.

In a basic overview for health professionals, Richards et al. (2016) defined non-binary and genderqueer genders and explored a variety of possible psychotherapeutic and biomedical interventions to affirm and support non-binary and genderqueer people in their gender experience. The medical and psychosocial intervention needs of non-binary and genderqueer individuals are diverse, and sensitivity to the needs of particular individuals is important (ibid.). Non-binary and genderqueer people routinely experience erasure in healthcare contexts, and feel forced to conform to binary gender narratives, even at specialty trans care clinics (Koehler, Eyssel and Nieder 2018; Lykens, LeBlanc and Bockting 2018; Taylor et al. 2019). The barriers to accessing gender-affirming medical care include systemic issues, incidents of bias, and insufficient medical provider education and awareness around the specific needs of trans and gender non-conforming people (Puckett et al. 2018). When clinicians misunderstand the different needs of gender diverse individuals, they risk collapsing people into binary trans identity categories, erasing their identities, and marginalizing them further. Academic research communities have committed the same error by collapsing non-binary, genderqueer, and other diverse LGBTQ identities into larger categories, thereby erasing them from data collection and analysis, despite these groups having unique health needs (Smalley, Warren and Barefoot 2016).

This erasure and marginalization occur on the wider social scale as well. Budge, Rossman, and Howard (2014) found that the genderqueer individuals they studied (N = 64) reported significantly higher anxiety and depres-

---

2   PubMed is an online database that aggregates health science articles and citations. It is maintained by the U.S. Library of Medicine and is visible at https://www.ncbi.nlm.nih.gov/pubmed/.

sion than in the general population and argued that this difference is due to being a stressed minority group rather than intrinsic pathology. Because non-binary and genderqueer people experience routine mis-gendering (e.g., strangers assuming a binary gender for them in speech and social assumptions), absence of media representation, pathologization, and social violence in the form of bullying and victimization, the experience of being genderqueer or non-binary can be stressful. Gender invalidation is a pervasive source of minority stress that affects non-binary individuals to a particularly significant degree (Johnson, LeBlanc, Deardorff and Bockting 2019). In addition to erasure and invalidation, victimization is a common experience for non-binary, genderqueer, and trans and gender non-conforming youth (Sterzing et al. 2017), and they report more risky behavior and experiences and fewer protective factors when compared with their cis gender peers (Eisenberg et al. 2017).

For professionals to help non-binary and genderqueer people navigate marginalizing social environments, it is helpful to provide supportive, culturally competent individual psychosocial support. In a chapter on psychotherapy with this population, Barker and Iantaffi (2017) give an overview of the challenges faced by these clients, examine the binarizing assumptions of different psychotherapeutic modalities, and enumerate likely gender-related issues that non-binary individuals may wish to examine in therapy. Rider et al. (2019) articulate a gender-affirmative lifespan approach (GALA) as a psychosocial intervention, which helps non-binary individuals build resiliency, develop gender literacy, move beyond the binary, promote positive sexuality, and move towards empowering medical interventions if desired. Interventions and therapeutic frameworks for helping non-binary and genderqueer people are beginning to appear, yet their wider dissemination and application is still very much needed.

Other authors have written clinical guides for psychotherapy with gender non-conforming children, youth and adults, with some attention to non-binary and genderqueer identities (Brill and Kenney 2016; Brill and Pepper 2008; Ehrensaft 2011; 2016; Keo-Meier and Ehrensaft 2018; Krieger 2017; Moe, Bower and Clark 2017). Others have published self-help workbooks for gender exploration and resilience (Bornstein 2006; 1998/2013; Hoffman-Fox 2017; Iantaffi and Barker 2017; Singh 2018; Testa, Coolhart and Peta 2015). Another important contribution is the publication of anthologies, first-person accounts and self-help guides that include theorized activism, such as Bornstein (1998/2013; 1994/2016), Bornstein and Bergman (2010), and Nestle, Howell and Wilchins

(2002). These short memoirs provide visibility, context, and a sense of community to those who are otherwise isolated and prevented from understanding their gender position due to an absence of narratives that explore, give words to, and validate the unique experiences of non-binary and genderqueer people.

Because social erasure and stigmatization play a key role in creating distress in non-binary individuals, it is crucial to foster cultural competence in healthcare. Interventions to support non-binary and genderqueer people are multileveled. Non-binary and genderqueer individuals need social support and help in adopting facilitative coping skills to navigate an overwhelmingly gender-binarizing world. Those who seek medical transition options need healthcare workers who can competently respond to their individual needs, rather than forcing them into a gender binarizing or trans-hostile medical paradigm. We also need to create broader change to foster a culture that acknowledges and celebrates gender diversity in all its forms, so as to counteract gender invalidation and cisheteronormativity. This chapter adds our voices to the call for greater acceptance, understanding, acknowledgement, support, and affirmation of our unique gender experiences.

Methods, Ethics, Recruitment, Data Collection

This pilot participatory action research study grew out of a non-binary/genderqueer peer support group in Portland, Oregon, USA which met twice a month from October 2016 to June 2017. The group was initially formed for community support, and as far as we know, ours was the first community group for non-binary and genderqueer people in Portland. The idea for this study came about after the group was well under way. We conducted this project as a participatory action research study (Brydon-Miller 1997), because we are all members of an oppressed group. We used a consensus-based model for making decisions, and the co-researchers were all invited to craft the shape of the research, produce data, and analyze it. Additionally, all the co-researchers have been invited to give feedback on the manuscript and include their names as co-authors.

Our aim in conducting this study was to increase cultural competency in counseling, with the specific goal of presenting our results at the Gender Odyssey Professional conference in Seattle, Washington, USA in August 2017. Because ours was a small study without institutional support, we con-

ducted an informal internal ethics review.[3] We determined to protect participant data through anonymity, and because we agreed to be co-researchers
together, we sought to reduce the risk of harm stemming from power dif-
ferentials. Based in our shared vision of activism, spreading awareness, and
sharing power, we felt that the traditional risks of power abuses stemming
from our research activities were minimal, and the potential for benefit from
publishing our results outweighed the risks of harm. As a small group of participant-members of an oppressed group who experience systemic marginalization and denial of access to resources, we hope that we can be trusted with
our own authority in choosing to publish the results of our findings on how
to treat non-binary and genderqueer people appropriately in counseling.

We recruited a convenience sample of support group members, our non-
binary and genderqueer friends, and past attendees. All past attendees were
emailed an invitation to two focus groups, held two weeks apart in June and
July 2017, which we held in the normal group meeting space (Sasha Strong's
psychotherapy office). Most of the in-person focus group co-researchers were
core members of the group; one of these individuals also participated in an
in-person informal interview at their home. Two other co-researchers sent
their accounts via email, and one of those individuals also participated in an
informal in-person interview at a restaurant. In all, our co-researchers (N =
7) included two mental health professionals, one primary care physician, two
K-12[4] educators, one educational para-professional, and one post-secondary
educator. Among us, we hold two doctoral degrees and four master's degrees.
Two of us are people of color, and the rest of us are white folks. Assigned
gender of birth data are omitted, as they are irrelevant for our purposes.

During the two focus groups, we discussed themes and experiences that
we thought were important, based on the following prompts:

"What has worked for you in therapy as a genderqueer/non-binary person?"
"What hasn't worked for you in therapy as a genderqueer/non-binary person?"

---

3   Of the two participant-researchers who had institutional affiliations at the time of the
     study, one worked at an institution that was hostile towards trans health issues, and
     the other institution had a policy not to offer institutional review board (IRB) review
     to students for projects not linked to doctoral theses. Due to these barriers, our study
     neither sought nor received formal IRB review.

4   In the U.S. education system, K-12 education refers to the compulsory educational pe-
     riod from kindergarten to grade 12, when students are between 5 and 18 years old.

"What other suggestions do you have for therapists to provide competent counseling services to genderqueer/non-binary people?"

During the focus groups, each co-researcher was invited to use standard U.S. format index cards[5] and write down significant themes, suggestions, and stories. After about 30 minutes (when the supply of cards was exhausted), we each read the contents of our cards and sorted them into themes (with each co-researcher having the final say in the goodness of fit of the theme to their data, and their data to the theme). Data collection and analysis happened incrementally and simultaneously, in a spiral of sampling and analysis (Creswell 2013). This process yielded 62 unique data items. These data were subsequently transcribed for clarity and posterity.[6]

Analysis

This project used a thematic analysis approach (Braun and Clarke 2006), We did not use a preexisting coding framework, but rather sought themes within the data. During the first focus group, we generated data and sorted cards into piles, coming up with 5 major themes. In the second focus group, we identified a need for concrete recommendations to improve clinical practice with non-binary and genderqueer folks. We gathered additional data on index cards, using the prompts "What are best practices for therapists working with genderqueer/non-binary clients?" and "What are poor practices for them?" During this time, we continued to practice a consensus-based thematic analysis method and implemented memoing and coding (Creswell 2013) of themes and best practices.

All participant-members of the focus groups were invited to join the core research group, but only two or three made it to subsequent planning meetings. During a meeting in mid-July 2017, we further refined the themes and entered additional data from an interview in a typewritten and index card format. At our next meeting in August 2017, two co-researchers (Sasha Strong and Sagan Wallace) further refined the Best Practices list and determined a

---

5   These paper cards measured 3x5 and 4x6 inches (roughly equivalent to A6 format) and were lined on one side.

6   Transcripts and data collection images are held by Sasha and are available to qualified researchers upon request for the purposes of study validation.

presentation format. Later in August 2017, Sasha & Sagan created a synopsis of the themes and prepared a bibliography for the conference handout. We presented at Gender Odyssey Professional[7] later that month to an interested audience of mental health professionals. Sagan has developed and offered presentations on their own to local universities and LGBTQ community groups. Sasha has presented to a few audiences of health professionals[8], has continued to develop the bibliography, and wrote this research report.

Results

Our study yielded five major themes and 12 best practices. The themes were Validation Basics, Holding Space for Complexity, Finding Safe Spaces, Erasure, and Trauma-Informed Intersectionality. The best practices appear after the presentation of themes below. The narrative text for each theme and best practice was written by Sasha and was developed from a global sense of the data we elicited. These sections extrapolate from the data to articulate how professionals can better meet our needs. Our findings are couched as imperatives, asking professionals to adapt their thinking and behavior to acknowledge, understand, and support our experience.

Validation Basics

The first major theme that should be taken into consideration when working with non-binary and genderqueer people is to validate our experience. It is hard to have a lived gender experience that is outside of the social norm, and we need people in our lives who will understand, affirm, and empathize with that experience. This does not necessarily mean that professionals need to have deep expertise on our identity, but just a basic sense of understanding our position and being willing to learn more in working with us.

We need to be validated as who we are. Please do not tell us to fit into a different identity, performance, or set of norms. Rather than policing our

---

7   Gender Odyssey is an annual U.S. West Coast conference on gender issues, first held in Seattle in 2001. We presented these findings in 2017 and 2018, in the professional track of the conference. Learn more at http://www.genderodyssey.org/.

8   A recording of one such presentation can be viewed at https://www.brilliancycounseli ng.com/blog/nbgq-counseling-competency-video/.

gender, please generate curiosity and appreciation for the richness of our gender diversity. While non-binary and genderqueer genders can be a bridge to other genders, they are also a location in their own right—telling us "it's just a phase" is profoundly insulting and misguided. Therefore, please refrain from undermining our identity with your assumptions, and please do not assume anything about our wishes, our medical needs, or our transition—just ask us!

Holding Space for Complexity

Non-binary and genderqueer experience are complex, mutable, and unfolds over time. We do not fit into the typical narratives of lifespan gender and identity development, and we may need to generate, revise, revisit, and recreate our gender identity, narrative, and path throughout life. Helping professionals who accompany us on this journey need to hold space for the complexity of this unfolding journey and encourage us to do the same. Helpers and companions who fearlessly nourish and encourage us during times of uncertainty are invaluable. Professionals who make gender assumptions that do not fit our experience, or who display discomfort with the ambiguity of our gender, risk damaging the therapeutic relationship and foreclosing the space of possibility.

Non-binary and genderqueer gender identity, performance, and development are complex, vary from person to person, and change over time. Our genders are as much about becoming as they are about being, and gender creativity begins with a sense of not-knowing and being willing to explore and find out. Non-binary and genderqueer people, and the people who support and help them, need to encourage gentle exploration with plenty of time to discover and create.

Finding Safe Spaces

Because we live in a cisheteronormative, gender binarizing culture, it is crucial for non-binary and genderqueer people to find safe spaces where we can feel validated, cared for, and understood. These spaces can occur in person, online, over the phone, or through books, websites, media, and other artifacts made by people like us. Just feeling that we are not alone is a crucial ingredient in helping us accept, love, and cherish ourselves and feel that we belong.

Safe spaces are needed everywhere, but especially when accessing services, in home life, with friends, and in the community. Peer support can be very helpful, especially in validating aspects of our experience that are misunderstood in other gendered contexts. When a safe space for our experience cannot be created, we appreciate referrals to competent counselors, community resources, and other non-binary/genderqueer-affirming groups and professionals.

Erasure

In the mainstream culture, our experience as non-binary and genderqueer people is characterized by repeated and pervasive erasure of our gender. Insomuch as gender is a core component of identity, basic facts about who we are get ignored and painted over all the time. Each time a stranger refers to us using a binary gender honorific or pronoun (e.g., Mr., Mrs., sir, madam, he, him, 'that guy'), or when a speaker addresses a group as "ladies and gentlemen," our identities are erased. People make binary gender assumptions constantly, and often, the result for us is pain and confusion. Whenever a stranger refrains from assigning us a binary gender identity in speech or manner, it can feel like a little victory of recognition—and yet it is just simple courtesy. Most of the time, strangers (and sometimes colleagues, friends, and family) erase us with their binary gender assumptions. Because this erasure is pervasive, and normative assumptions about binary genders mostly go unquestioned in mainstream social discourse, it is crucial that helpers understand this pain, and that they not recapitulate it.

Trauma-Informed Intersectionality

Crenshaw (1989) discussed how multiple intersecting aspects of identity come together to create unique configurations of social identity and oppression, in a theory that has come to be called "intersectionality." Along with an acknowledgement of the complexity of our identities (which may also include racialized identities, disability-related identities, different countries of origin, socialized genders, etc.) comes an acknowledgement that social oppression can contribute to trauma. Many of us have experienced trauma, and while our non-binary/genderqueer experience intersects with trauma and may be entangled with its aftereffects, our trauma does not cause our non-binary/genderqueer gender, and our gender does not cause our trauma. Those who claim that trauma causes gender difference, commit a profoundly pathologizing error, and they do epistemological and social violence to a person's gender location and lived experience as a survivor of trauma. That said, supportive, trauma-informed services that are non-pathologizing and strengths-based can be helpful in addressing the biographical trauma we have experienced, as well as the repeated and pervasive social trauma we experience due to our gender difference and other oppressed social group memberships. We need competent professionals who can approach this complex interrelationship with sensitivity and discernment.

12 Best Practices

The following statements are written to address health providers, but they can also serve as points of reflection for non-binary, genderqueer, and gender diverse people to understand their own experience, as well as to advocate for their needs in healthcare and other contexts.

1. Embrace gender transition as an open-ended, lifelong process of exploration and joy. There is no timeline, correct answer, or final destination for the gender journey. Rather, it is an open field of play.

2. Be curious about NB/GQness in general and the unique experience of individuals in particular. Non-binary and genderqueer experience are improvisational, innovative, and open to constant discovery. When you bring your curiosity, it synergizes with our experience to promote optimal gender exploration and growth.

3. Don't use your clients for your professional education. Rather, read up, network with competent peers, and attend trainings. Certainly, individuals are experts on their own experience, but if you need more education on the generalities of non-binary and genderqueer issues, please consult the bibliography, engage in continuing education opportunities, or contact the authors for training and consultation.

4. Get our pronouns right (and if you mess up, apologize, and move on). Different people use different pronouns at different times for different reasons. The most polite approach is to ask a person what pronouns they use the first time you meet them, do your best to observe those preferences, and accept corrections and revisions in the future. If you erroneously misgender someone by using the wrong pronoun (or another gendered word) and notice your mistake, simply apologize sincerely, and move on to the next thing. Kindly refrain from long-winded, over-dramatic apologies that make of us the victims and caretakers of your social anxiety and awkwardness.

5. Appreciate the rich complexity of transness. The trans umbrella is big enough to fit all the people whose gender transcends cis and/or binary genders. Please develop an appreciation for this richness, and for all the ways that people choose to live and perform their genders. Isn't it wonderful that there are so many ways to be human? Gender is a category of expression that allows for endless creativity.

6. Start from within: Analyze your own gender assumptions, limitations, and position(s). After learning to refrain from misgendering us, perhaps the next best step is to analyze and deconstruct your own gender socialization. By analyzing your own gender position and understanding the ways that power, privilege, and oppression run through it, you can reduce your discomfort when you meet someone who challenges your gender assumptions. By doing your own gender work, you reduce the risk harming others by reflexively and unreflectively enforcing cisheteropatriarchy and your gender socialization. Guidebooks to this process can be helpful (e.g., Iantaffi and Barker 2017; Bornstein 1998/2013), as can discussing your experience with competent friends.

7. Change your intake forms, policies, and processes to avoid binary gender assumptions. While insurance companies and other institutions may still require binary gender markers for reimbursement purposes, you can probably change pretty much every other aspect of your administrative environment to include and support gender non-conforming people. Donatone and Rachlin (2013) described how they created psychotherapy intake templates that are inclusive of trans identities. Remember that physical anatomy, names, pronouns, gender, romantic/affective attraction, and sexual attraction are independent dimensions that constellate differently for different people (Bornstein 1998/2013; Pan, Moore and Trans Student Educational Resources, n.d.). Please adjust your procedures and policies with those realities in mind.

8. Change your speech to avoid binary gender assumptions. The linguistic practice of assuming and imposing binary genders is only a habit, and just like any other habit, it can be unlearned and reshaped. When addressing strangers or speaking to someone about a person you don't know, refrain from assuming you know the gender of the person. For example, rather than saying "that man over there," use a non-gendered way to clarify who you mean, such as "the person in the green shirt." This helps in practicing a new habit, and it models communication outside an assumed gender binary to those you are speaking with. Likewise, in addressing clients, patients, and students, find ways to abstain from imposing binary gender assumptions on them and on the people, you talk about (if their genders are unknown). Although English lacks clear gender-neutral honorific forms, it is possible to avoid most other gender-binarizing formulations; other languages may present different degrees of ease and challenge. These practices extend into written communications and go a long way to help non-binary and genderqueer people feel understood and respected—simply by avoiding common practices that marginalize us and erase our experience and existence.

9. Develop a relationship with the community that goes beyond learning from us. Making friends, volunteer work, and supporting artistic and cultural productions by non-binary and genderqueer people are a few ways to build full human relationships with us.

10. Understand that trauma and non-binary/genderqueer experience co-arise and are intertwined, but one does not cause the other. This major theme bears repeating as a best practice. Trauma does not make us non-binary or genderqueer, and our gender identity does not cause our psychological trauma. Just as trauma can arise and interact with any other intersectional identity, our non-binary/genderqueer gender is one among many aspects of who are.

11. Develop a critical analysis of systems of oppression and intersectionality. Gender, transphobia, cisheteronormativity, and violence against gender non-conforming people are all parts of an interlinked chain of privilege, oppression, and violence that are inseparable from capitalism, white supremacy, the military-industrial complex, and the school-to-prison pipeline. If you genuinely analyze the profound injustices of our current social system and come to understand how these injustices are created, perpetuated, and enforced, you will be able to use your positionality and privilege to interrupt these processes of injustice and promote the welfare of non-binary and genderqueer people—and indeed everyone who experiences identity-based oppression in our shared world.

12. Carry forth these principles and become a non-binary/genderqueer ally and activist!
Please join us in doing this work—we need as many allies and activists as possible. If you do choose to join us, please be willing continually to examine your gender, your positionality, and your privilege, in order to reduce unintended harm and to promote the welfare of all. We want to welcome you and celebrate your creativity, contributions, resilience, and courage, as you welcome us and celebrate ours.

Limitations and Discussion

This study was conducted with a small number of participants and may not be generalizable to other populations. However, qualitative studies do not aim for statistical generalizability (Tracy 2010), and these data are an initial step in asking the experts—non-binary and genderqueer people—what they need from counselors and, by extension, other helping professionals. Our findings resonate with the clinical guidelines and qualitative results of other authors (e.g., Barker and Iantaffi 2017; Richards et al. 2016; Rider et al. 2019; Taylor et al. 2019), and such resonance lends credence to our claims. Future studies could validate and expand on our findings.

Because our project seeks to influence helping professionals to attend to our needs as non-binary and genderqueer individuals, the data we elicited is biased towards our desire to persuade helpers to meet our perceived needs and create cultural change. A desired social outcome is a feature of participatory action research (Brydon-Miller 1997). As our research group included two mental health professionals, four educators, and one primary care physician, we feel that we are relatively knowledgeable about the needs of non-binary and genderqueer people in these contexts, and what our colleagues could do to learn more to support non-binary and genderqueer individuals. I, Sasha, trust that the research group's contextually grounded understanding of our most pressing communal concerns is an appropriate guide for bringing forth the most important aspects of these data. We are the experts on our own experience.

While we have applied thematic analysis as a qualitative research method (Braun and Clarke 2006) and brought critical gender theories to bear in terms of understanding our own experiences of gender and their intersections with other oppressed social identities (e.g., Bornstein 1998/2013; Butler 1999/2006), our research strategy is fundamentally a participatory action research project which has valorized first-person experience and expertise, consensus-based decision-making, and improved outcomes for non-binary and genderqueer people (Brydon-Miller 1997). Our overt activist goals may make our project seem less 'objective' by traditional academic standards. However, we feel that research grounded in critical emancipatory values is more appropriate for this topic than research that feigns neutrality but favors and recapitulates hidden axiological assumptions of dominance and control. Guba and Lincoln (1994) articulated competing paradigmatic assumptions of qualitative and quantitative research and critiqued the implicit values of quantitative research. Our value commitments in this study are that we matter, and we would like to help professionals to do a better job. Please do not erase or devalue our voices because the knowledge we present here does not look like the kind of science which exemplifies the 'disembodied white cis male expert' approach. That said, we welcome sincere critical engagement with our research.

We have no funders or publication requirements for tenure, so our work does not conform to those pressures. Rather, our aim is to promote the welfare and opportunities of non-binary and genderqueer people and educate professionals through this work. We hope that you, the reader, will believe that this study articulates the changes we would like you to make in your healthcare practice, so as to acknowledge and accommodate us. Our expertise on these matters comes from our own lived experience.

We recruited using a convenience and snowball sample, based on our support group members and their friends, and we did not attempt to recruit a larger sample. One could challenge our truth claims based on this sampling procedure, but we believe that our findings remain valid despite the small size of the sample. One could also critique the sample because we came together for mutual support and created friendships and camaraderie through this process. Such a critique assumes that genuine human relationships somehow hinder the acquisition of knowledge. To assume that individuals from an oppressed group need to adopt a set of values and procedures that are impersonal, disconnected, and politically neutral is to impose white cisheteropatriarchal values upon queer, non-binary, racially diverse individuals. There are many kinds of knowing and coming to know oneself through social connection is of significant value in building understanding and resilience for oppressed groups (Nieto et al. 2014). In this sense, the support group sensitized research group members to the needs discussed in the study, because for many of us, it was the first time we came together with other non-binary and genderqueer individuals in a group setting over a long period. If one has a need that has never been met, and then one is able to meet it by spending time with alike individuals, it becomes possible to articulate that need in a way that was impossible before (ibid.). Our findings and this paper are an outcome of the resilience we built and experienced together; we are happy to share it.

Methodologically, one could challenge the validity of our results by saying that we did not achieve saturation of the categories.[9] However, we are not trying to articulate all of the ways that professional helpers should change their practices to meet our needs; rather we hope to provide good initial guidance. We also hope that interested readers will deepen their learning on this topic in the future.

Tracy (2010) articulated eight big-tent criteria for quality in qualitative research, and my sense is that this study addresses a worthy topic; achieves sincerity, credibility, resonance, and meaningful coherence; and makes a significant contribution. Tracy's (2010) criterion of rich rigor would be better supported by exposing more of the specific data points in this study. However, we have chosen not to do so in order to protect the anonymity of our co-researchers. I, Sasha, believe that the themes and best practices we elicited make sense of our experience in a way that accurately communicates information about our needs to our intended audience in a salient way. We welcome future studies that will validate, deepen, or dispute our findings.

As to Tracy's (2010) ethical criterion for qualitative research, this study conducted a semi-formal internal ethics procedure, in which we sought consent and consensus from research group members during the study. This included contextual and procedural ethics relating to the comfort and preferences of our co-researchers. While we did not seek IRB approval, our internal process has included consensual decision-making in the research process and consideration of the risk of harm and the potential for benefit in conducting and publishing this study. All seven research group members were invited to share authorship, but only four responded to emailed invitations.

While a few works in our bibliography were discovered by research group members in their search for self-understanding and affirmation prior to the study, the formal literature search was completed after data collection and analysis occurred. It simply seemed unwieldy to ask our co-researchers, most

---

9   Theoretical saturation was first introduced in the grounded theory method of qualitative research (Glaser & Strauss, 1967), but it is not an appropriate standard for all qualitative approaches (O'Reilly & Parker, 2013).

of whom are not academics, to conduct a literature review prior to participating in the study. As our data and categories emerged from our lived experiences foremost, they are unlikely to be predetermined or influenced by existing research findings. That said, many of the themes and best practices we discovered are echoed in the literature reviewed above, and this form of triangulation lends credence to our claims.

This study elicited suggestions for how to improve counseling for non-binary and genderqueer people, and I (Sasha) believe that these findings are generalizable to other healthcare contexts, such as medicine. While articles from those fields lend support to this argument (e.g., Koehler, Eyssel and Nieder 2018; Lykens, LeBlanc and Bockting 2018; Puckett et al. 2018; Smalley, Warren and Barefoot 2016; Sterzing et al. 2017; Taylor et al. 2019), more studies asking non-binary and genderqueer individuals about their needs in healthcare are required.

Conclusion

Counselors, mental health professionals, and other healthcare providers are uniquely poised to foster supportive environments for non-binary and genderqueer people. Our hope is that you will take our recommendations to heart and begin to change your own relationship to the gender binary so as to validate us, hold space for complexity with us as we develop, create safe spaces, erase us less, approach any trauma in our past with respect and sensitivity, and adopt the 12 best practices we recommend above. Thank you for caring about us!

References

Barker, M.J. and Iantaffi, A. (2017): Psychotherapy. In: Richards, C.; Bouman, W.P. and Barker, M.J. (Eds.): Genderqueer and non-binary genders. New York: Palgrave Macmillan, pp. 103-124.

Bornstein, K. (2006): Hello, cruel world: 101 alternatives to suicide for teens, freaks, and other outlaws. New York: Seven Stories Press.

Bornstein, K. (2013): My new gender workbook: A step-by-step guide to achieving world peace through gender anarchy and sex positivity (2nd ed.). New York: Routledge (Original work published 1998).

Bornstein, K. (2016): Gender outlaw: On men, women, and the rest of us (2nd rev. ed.). New York: Vintage Books (Original work published 1994).

Bornstein, K. and Bergman, S.B. (Eds.) (2010): Gender outlaws: The next generation (Reprint ed.). Berkeley: Seal Press.

Braun, V. and Clarke, V. (2006): Using thematic analysis in psychology. In: Qualitative Research in Psychology, 3(2), pp. 77–101.

Brill, S.A. and Kenney, L. (2016): The transgender teen: A handbook for parents and professionals supporting transgender and non-binary teens. San Francisco: Cleis Press.

Brill, S.A. and Pepper, R. (2008): The transgender child: A handbook for families and professionals. San Francisco: Cleis Press.

Brydon-Miller, M. (1997): Participatory Action Research: Psychology and social change. In: Journal of Social Issues, 53(4), pp. 657–666.

Budge, S.L.; Rossman, H.K. and Howard, K.A.S. (2014): Coping and psychological distress among genderqueer individuals: The moderating effect of social support. In: Journal of LGBT Issues in Counseling, 8(1), pp. 95–117.

Butler, J. (2006): Gender trouble: Feminism and the subversion of identity. New York: Routledge (Original work published 1999).

Crenshaw, K. (1989): Demarginalizing the intersection of race and sex: A Black Feminist critique of antidiscrimination doctrine, feminist theory and antiracist politics. In: University of Chicago Legal Forum, 1989(1), pp. 139–167.

Creswell, J.W. (2013): Qualitative Inquiry and Research Design: Choosing Among Five Traditions (3rd ed.). Thousand Oaks: SAGE Publications.

Donatone, B. and Rachlin, K. (2013): An intake template for transgender, transsexual, genderqueer, gender nonconforming, and gender variant college students seeking mental health services. In: Journal of College Student Psychotherapy, 27(3), pp. 200–211.

Ehrensaft, D. (2011): Gender born, gender made: Raising healthy gender-nonconforming children (3rd rev. ed.). New York: The Experiment.

Ehrensaft, D. (2016): The gender creative child: Pathways for nurturing and supporting children who live outside gender boxes. New York: The Experiment.

Eisenberg, M.E.; Gower, A.L.; McMorris, B.J., Rider, G.N.; Shea, G. and Coleman, E. (2017): Risk and protective factors in the lives of transgender/gender nonconforming adolescents. In: Journal of Adolescent Health, 61(4), pp. 521–526.

Glaser, B.G. and Strauss, A.L. (1967): The discovery of grounded theory: Strategies for qualitative research. New York: AldineTransaction.

Guba, E.G. and Lincoln, Y.S. (1994): Competing paradigms in qualitative research. In: Denzin, N.K. and Lincoln, Y.S. (Eds.): Handbook of qualitative research. Thousand Oaks: Sage, pp. 105-117.

Hoffman-Fox, D. (2017): You and your gender identity: A guide to discovery. New York: Skyhorse.

Iantaffi, A. and Barker, M.J. (2017): How to understand your gender: A practical guide for exploring who you are. London: Jessica Kingsley Publishers.

James, S.E.; Herman, J.L.; Rankin, S.; Keisling, M.; Mottet, L. and Anafi, M. (2016). The report of the 2015 U.S. Transgender Survey. National Center for Transgender Equality [online]. Washington, DC: National Center for Transgender Equality. Available at: https://transequality.org/sites/def ault/files/docs/usts/USTS-Full-Report-Dec17.pdf (Accessed: 04 December 2021).

Keo-Meier, C. and Ehrensaft, D. (Eds.) (2018): The gender affirmative model: An interdisciplinary approach to supporting transgender and gender expansive children. Washington, DC: American Psychological Association.

Koehler, A.; Eyssel, J. and Nieder, T.O. (2018): Genders and individual treatment progress in (non-)binary trans individuals. In: The Journal of Sexual Medicine, 15(1), pp. 102–113.

Krieger, I. (2017): Counseling transgender and non-binary youth: The essential guide. London: Jessica Kingsley Publishers.

Lykens, J.E.; LeBlanc, A.J. and Bockting, W.O. (2018): Healthcare experiences among young adults who identify as genderqueer or nonbinary. LGBT Health, 5(3), pp. 191–196.

Nieto, L., Boyer, M.F.; Goodwin, L.; Johnson, G.R.; Smith, L.C. and Hopkins, J.P. (2014): Beyond inclusion, beyond empowerment: A developmental strategy to liberate everyone. Olympia: Cuetzpalin.

Moe, J.; Bower, J. and Clark, M. (2017): Counseling queer and genderqueer people. In: Ginicola, M.M.; Smith, C. and Filmore, J.M. (Eds.): Affirmative counseling with LGBTQI+ people. Alexandria: American Counseling Association, pp. 213-226.

Nestle, J.; Howell, C. and Wilchins, R.A. (Eds.) (2002): Genderquakes: Voices from beyond the sexual binary. Los Angeles: Alyson Books.

O'Reilly, M. and Parker, N. (2013): 'Unsatisfactory Saturation': A critical exploration of the notion of saturated sample sizes in qualitative research. In: Qualitative Research, 13(2), pp. 190–197.

Pan, L.; Moore, A. and Trans Student Educational Resources. (n.d.): The gender unicorn [online]. Available at: https://transstudent.org/gender/ (Accessed: 04 December 2021).

Puckett, J.A.; Cleary, P.; Rossman, K.; Mustanski, B. and Newcomb, M.E. (2018): Barriers to gender-affirming care for transgender and gender nonconforming individuals. In: Sexuality Research and Social Policy, 15(1), pp. 48–59.

Richards, C.; Bouman, W.P. and Barker, M.J. (2017): Genderqueer and non-binary genders. New York: Palgrave Macmillan.

Richards, C.; Bouman, W.P.; Seal, L.; Barker, M.J.; Nieder, T.O. and T'Sjoen, G. (2016): Non-binary or genderqueer genders. In: International Review of Psychiatry, 28(1), pp. 95–102.

Rider, G.N.; Vencill, J.A.; Berg, D.R.; Becker-Warner, R.; Candelario-Pérez, L. and Spencer, K.G. (2019): The gender affirmative lifespan approach (GALA): A framework for competent clinical care with nonbinary clients. In: International Journal of Transgenderism, 20(2–3), pp. 275–288.

Singh, A.A. (2018): The queer and transgender resilience workbook: Skills for navigating sexual orientation and gender expression. Oakland: New Harbinger Publications Inc.

Smalley, K.B.; Warren, J.C. and Barefoot, K.N. (2016): Differences in health risk behaviors across understudied LGBT subgroups. In: Health Psychology, 35(2), pp. 103–114.

Sterzing, P.R.; Ratliff, G.A.; Gartner, R.E.; McGeough, B.L. and Johnson, K.C. (2017): Social ecological correlates of polyvictimization among a national sample of transgender, genderqueer, and cisgender sexual minority adolescents. In: Child Abuse & Neglect, 67, pp. 1–12.

Taylor, J.; Zalewska, A.; Gates, J.J. and Millon, G. (2019): An exploration of the lived experiences of non-binary individuals who have presented at a gender identity clinic in the United Kingdom. In: International Journal of Transgenderism, 20(2–3), pp. 195–204.

Testa, R.J.; Coolhart, D. and Peta, J. (2015). The gender quest workbook: A guide for teens & young adults exploring gender identity. Oakland: Instant Help Books.

Tracy, S.J. (2010): Qualitative quality: Eight "big-tent" criteria for excellent qualitative research. In: Qualitative Inquiry, 16(10), pp. 837–851.

Trans in Practice, Transition in Sequence: Providing Medical Assistance for Gender Transitions in Trans and Gender Non-Conforming Youth

Jeremy Gottlieb

Each clinical visit at the pediatric gender clinic begins with three knocks. After a sharp rap on the closed door, the pediatric endocrinologist pushes the handle and enters the consultation room without hesitation. From there, a world of possibilities opens. This paper explores the possibilities these clinic-room doors open.

Biomedicine has been 'treating' trans adults in the United States with hormones since Harry Benjamin championed endocrine therapy in the 1950s (Benjamin 1954). Children and adolescents, on the other hand, have only recently become eligible for transition related medical intervention. It was not until 2009 that the "Endocrine Society" first recommended puberty blockers as part of "treatment of transsexual" children (Hembree et al. 2009; Gill-Peterson 2018).[1] This medical care has been impactful for trans young people, who experience disproportionate levels of mental health issues (Becerra-Culqui et al. 2018) and homelessness (Whitbeck et al. 2014) compared with cis-gender youth. In 2019, the state of Minnesota in the US found that "transgender students in the 11th grade... are more than four times more likely to attempt suicide than their cisgender 11th-grade peers" (Minnesota Department of Health 2019). In aggregate, trans youth face a 41 percent lifetime suicide attempt risk (Haas, Rodgers and Herman 2014), as compared to a 3.0-5.1 per-

---

1   The "Endocrine Society" is the leading professional medical organization for endocrinology in the United States. It publishes standards and recommendations for care of endocrine conditions, as well as hormone management for trans individuals.

cent lifetime suicide attempt rate in the general US population (Nock et al. 2008).

It is under this shadow of transphobia and trans youth suicide that I conducted ethnographic fieldwork within a pediatric gender clinic in the United States for 5 months in 2017 through 2018. Drawing on this ethnographic data, I will first briefly explore the ontology of gender and transness within a pediatric gender clinic, and then employ this understanding to examine the temporal sequence of transition within the gender clinic. I draw on Annemarie Mol's work, *The Body Multiple* (2002), to explore how gender is enacted in practice and how multiple enactments of gender interact to bring realities of trans people into being (see Latham 2017 for a trans autoethnographic engagement with Mol's work). I employ Mol's term, "enacted," because in the gender clinic actions are occurring that bring gender and transness to the forefront and into being. Gender and transness are not simply known; they are *done*. Per Mol's application, enactment implies that "objects [genders] come into being—and disappear—with the practices in which they are manipulated" (Mol 2002:5). Enactment "suggests that activities take place... [and] that in the act, and only then and there, something *is*—being enacted" (ibid.:33). In the practices of the gender clinic an ontology of gender and transness arises.[2]

After establishing this ontological claim, I expand the focus of this essay to unpack how enactments of gender are temporally structured in the creation of a transition. Specifically, I name three relationships of enactments—predication, obstruction, and justification—which sequence realities of gender and transness. These relationships, respectively, form, disrupt, or accelerate the normative sequence of transition enforced by biomedicine within the gender clinic.

I conclude the paper by acknowledging the utilitarian value of the gender clinic's normative sequence, while exploring the ways an understanding of gender and trans ontologies and their sequencing can improve and expand the care of trans youth beyond biomedicine's enforced normative sequence of transition.

---

2   This is true for cis- as well as trans people. A separate ethnography could explore the how gender is enacted throughout clinics not specifically designed for trans patients. The practices of medicine bring gender – and its many ontologies – into being in these spaces.

Trans in Practice

In *The Body Multiple* (2002), Annemarie Mol traces atherosclerosis and its many ontologies through a Dutch hospital. She argues that atherosclerosis is "enacted" differently by patients, surgeons, doctors, nurses, and varying medical technologies. Accordingly, the ontological reality of what atherosclerosis *is* multiplies.

Transness is likewise *done* in multiple ways by and with numerous actors in the gender clinic. Yet gender and transness as ontology are also unruly. Their multiple realities – the multiple ways of enacting gender and transness – sometimes align, but often conflict or take precedence over one another. And for a child in transition, the socio-material practices of the clinic, as well as the ways the child moves through the gendered world outside of the clinic, offer many modes in which gender and transness can be done and undone.

To understand the multiple ontologies of transness, one must consider the diverse realities of gender and the practices that realize their being. This is essential, of course, because gender is what is being 'trans-d' in the pediatric gender clinic. While I argue transness is brought into being in the conflict of gender enactments, the object brought into being, transness, is not a botched gender or a failure to fit into the order of things. Rather, transness appears in the conflict of gender enactments as something greater than the dissonant gender enactments. Put differently, 'trans-ing' gender creates an object that is more than just normative gender. To understand this, lets return to those three knocks:

Three short knocks and the doctor strides into the last consult of her day. Khalif, a young child dressed in baggy jeans and an orange t-shirt, is just climbing off the exam table.

> *"How are we doing today?" the doctor asks, both as a pleasantry and a coded way to ask 'what brings you in?'*
> *"We're doing well," Khalif's mom replies, "Khalif came into his kindergarten socially transitioned. He wears boy clothes and likes his hair cut as a Mohawk."*
> *The doctor turns from her computer to Khalif and asks, "And Khalif, what pronouns do you use?"*
> *"He," Khalif answers quietly, lowering his gaze sheepishly to his swinging feet.*
> *"Well, I use she, her, hers, [myself]," the doctor says kindly. "How has school been?"*
> *"Good," Khalif again says quietly.*

"Good," Khalif's mom echoes, "All of the teachers know Khalif is trans and are sup-
portive. They use his correct name and his pronouns. We haven't had any problems
with any of the other kids." As the endocrinologist gets up and starts washing her
hands, the mom goes on: "I'm in an online support group for parents with trans kids
and I wanted to come in today because I want to know a timeline of when we should
start Khalif on [puberty] blockers and T[estosterone]."

The doctor begins her normal check-up routine: moving her stethoscope along the
Khalif's chest and back as he breathes, shining a light into his eyes, ears, and mouth.
She explains that she starts her patients on blockers when the child begins puberty.
Hormone replacement therapy [HRT] normally starts at 16 years old at the earliest,
but if "we know the child is trans, we can start hormones earlier."

Khalif's mom and I both sit silently as the doctor continues with her exam. She
checks Khalif's armpits for hair, his chest for any breast tissue growth, and com-
pletes a genital exam.

To end the consult, the endocrinologist explains the different ways blockers can be
administered — injections, pill, or patch — and tells Khalif and his mom to return in a
year or if they start to see any signs of puberty. "Look for breast tissue development
first. That could start around age nine." [3]

Gender is done in many different ways in this consultation. Khalif's male
identity is enacted as wearing clothes associated with boys, his Mohawk hair-
cut, and the pronouns he uses. The doctor might describe Khalif's maleness
as a lack of breast development. In Khalif's case, we see his gender is done
through multiple registers: style, language, the body, and by various people:
his mom and teachers, Khalif himself, the doctor in the clinic. I argue Khalif's
male gender is multiple because pronouns are not a lack of breast tissue,
which are also not haircuts. Yet gender is all of these things. This is what
it means to hold Khalif's male gender as multiple.

However, 'boy' is not the only gender identity brought into being in
Khalif's clinical visit. When the endocrinologist turns to Khalif's medical file,
she sees Khalif's legal, female name and an 'F' standing under the category of
sex, imported from Khalif's state-issued birth certificate. Likewise, female is
enacted in the doctor's visual assessment of Khalif's vagina, and her palpation

---

3   I was able to observe clinical visits at the pediatric gender clinic after receiving IRB
     approval from the clinic's hospital and informed consent from the providers. Informed
     consent was obtained from patients if they were over 18 years old and from patients'
     parents/guardians with the patient's assent if the patient was under 18 years old for all
     interviews.

of his breast tissue. In fact, temporal ruptures bring many of these female enactments into the present. The 'F' on Khalif's birth certificate (a state and institutional enactment of gender) is dragged from the past into the medical record while a future referential of breast development is brought across Khalif's body and into the exam room through the doctor's breast exam.[4]

Transness is brought into being when these enactments of 'female' are held against the realities of stereotypical masculinity also present in the consultation room. Trans materializes when Khalif's legal name stands next to 'he' and when the doctor discusses chemicals that will foreclose a particular form of bodily development. Trans is enacted when the 'F' on Khalif's birth certificate ruptures into the present and stands next to his male enactments of hair and clothing styles. Without this encounter between male and female enactments, trans would not come into being in the gender clinic. Khalif enacts 'boyness' until the doctor examines his chest and genitals or looks through his medical file. It is only then that trans is brought into being. Trans is enacted by practices over and over again in the gender clinic. Gender enactments such as the speech act, "I am a boy," haircuts, blood tests for hormone levels, teste size, deepening voices, 'peach fuzz' above the lip, and menses are held against one another as well as past and future enactments to bring transness into being.

Transition in Sequence

Foregrounding the practices of the gender clinic reveals that gender comes into being in socio-material practices. Trans ontology, in turn, is enacted as these practices are held against one another. I now wish to explore how relationships between enactments of gender and trans bring about a transition within the pediatric gender clinic.

---

4   Many of the practices of the gender clinic queer time. For instance, in Khalif's case, both past and present appear in the present. Similarly, abstracting the term "chrononormativity" from Elizabeth Freeman's *Time Binds* (2010), we can see how the gender clinic's interventions queer the chrononormative timeline of development put forward by western medicine. Many of the gender clinic's patients go through a second puberty, or blockers will cause a "temporal drag," in which prepubescence is maintained for years beyond it's 'normal' expected conclusion (Freeman 2010). This is what Lauren Berlant would describe as an "impasse" (Berlant 2011), and Kathryn Bond Stockton would argue is "growing sideways" (Stockton 2009).

The pediatric gender clinic's intervention orients itself around transition; the endocrinologist tells me, "As the endocrinologist what I'm trying to do is to help their bodies align more with their gender identity." Consequently, the gender clinic is as much about gender identity as it is about development, about change over and through time. The relationship between enactments of gender and transness reveals sequences that define development and transition. Certain forms of development will stall while others will proceed. And, critically, when one analyzes the temporal relationships between gender and trans enactments in the clinic, certain epistemological assumptions about transitions and development arise. Succinctly, the gender clinic imagines and enacts a normative time(line) of transition. Certain enactments of gender are necessary for the sequence of transition to proceed, others block the sequence from advancing, and still others move the sequence along at a faster rate than the 'normal' trans subject or the 'normal' sequence. I will call these relationships predication, obstruction, and justification, respectively.

Predication is that relationship in which an enactment must be done, must be present, for a sequence to proceed. For instance, a letter of support from a psychotherapist is required to predicate a medical intervention. The enactment of gender as a letter of support must precede enactments such as hormone levels, breast development, or voice deepening. Predication is the foundation of the sequence. It can be thought of as a check point, a necessary step.

Obstruction is the relationship of enactments that foreclose other enactments from coming into being or completely shields them from view. It occurs when enactments inhibit the sequence of transition from proceeding and thus occlude certain enactments of gender and transness from coming into being. This reveals contesting sequences of transition (some of which are the absence of a transition) and how certain enactments can produce violence against trans subjects.

Lastly, justification is an accelerant. In contrast to obstructions, which hamper or terminate a transition, these enactments bring others into being, pull them into the sequence, before they would normally occur. As revealed by Khalif's visit, the endocrinologist 'normally' begins HRT at sixteen years old. However, if the gender clinic "knows the child is trans" hormones can be administered starting at fifteen. As I will discuss, the enactment of the gender clinic 'knowing' a patient is trans accelerates the normative sequence and allows the patient to enact gender as hormones (and changing body fat distribution, etc.) earlier than sixteen.

These relationships – predication, obstruction, and justification – are an organizing schema, but they are not meant to imply there is no grey area or overlap between them. It is possible that enactments of gender and transness may fall into multiple categories or somewhere in between. For instance, a letter of support predicates other (medical) enactments; however, withholding a letter is a form of obstruction. Likewise, the opposite of many obstructions may sometimes (often when massively combined) act as accelerants to a transition. Finally, a second way to think about these terms is what these relationships mean for sequence. Thus, one can also read this schema: normative sequence, dissonance within the sequence, and accelerants of the sequence.

Many enactments of gender within the gender clinic can be temporally unregimented and diverse. A patient does not need to legally change their name, or go by a chosen name at all, before the patient injects a hormone into their body. While hairstyles, chest binders, and makeup all bring gender into being, none must precede or follow another. There is no strict temporal linearity or sequence to these events in the gender clinic. However, a letter of support from a mental health provider must always predicate any medical intervention from the clinic (Hembree et al. 2017). In requiring this predicative relationship between a letter of support and levels of hormones within one's blood, a sequence emerges.

> Logan is in his mid-teens when I meet him. His hair is colored a mélange of blue, grey and purple. When the social worker tells Logan he's now ready for testosterone, a smile arches across his face that will stay with him for the rest of the visit. "We do need a letter of support, though," the social worker says. "How is therapy going?" she then asks.
>
> "It's good. I don't like the group sessions much, but I can go to more of the group therapy if that means I can get a letter of support," Logan replies, not letting this roadblock temper his excitement.
>
> "Who's your mental health provider, again?" the clinical social worker asks rhetorically as she looks down at her notes. "Ah! Well, I can also give you a referral to one of the gender friendly mental health providers we recommend. I do want you to keep going to group therapy, but we need that letter before we can start you on T. I'll tell you what, though, let me go talk to the doctor and we can probably send you the prescription for T once we get that letter, so you don't have to wait until your next visit."

As the first checkpoint in the standard timeline of transition, scenes of acquiring a letter of support in order to begin medical treatment at the gender clinic happen often. One mother tries to get her son's psychologist on the phone while she and her son are still in the clinical consult. Another patient had completed a round of therapy before they came to the gender clinic, but learned they need to return to a psychotherapist in order to obtain a letter of support.

Logan's consultation and many others reveal the predicative role of the psychotherapist's letter of support to gender enacted as hormones or puberty blockers. Moreover, one observes a normative sequence unfolding. First a letter, then hormones. To bring gender as hormones or blockers (the lack of hormones) into being, transness enacted as a diagnosis of gender dysphoria must be present.

The gender clinic premises its medical intervention on the letter of support in order to meet the medical standards of care set by *the World Professional Association for Transgender Health (WPATH)* and the "Endocrine Society" (Coleman et al. 2012; Hembree et al. 2017). One of the criteria for a "physical intervention" in these standards of care is that adolescents must demonstrate gender non-conformity and gender dysphoria. This standard is in place to make sure the medical apparatus does not complete a "physical intervention" when in fact a patient does not desire a "physical intervention." However, this same safety, or check, is not applied to the endocrinologist's other pediatric endocrinology patients. For instance, the doctor describes a cis gender patient in her general pediatric endocrinology clinic, who is frustrated that he has not begun puberty. It turns out that he has a hormonal disorder in which he is not producing (enough) sex hormones. Consequently, the endocrinologist prescribes him testosterone. What is important to note here is that the patient does not need a letter of support from a mental health professional verifying his distress in order to receive medical care.

This cis male patient had to give informed consent with his parents, a standard of ethics in western medicine. So, too, do the patients in the gender clinic. However, the requirement of trans patients to acquire a letter of support in addition to their consent before a medical intervention reveals a socio-medical doubt of their transness. Trans patients are required to obtain a letter of support in order to *prove* their identity. Cis patients visiting the pediatric endocrinology clinic do not need to prove their distress with a psychological acknowledgement that a lack of medical care will maintain their suffering. They are taken at face value.

The necessary predication of a letter of support to the clinic's intervention forces the pediatric trans patient to fall into an enforced normative sequence.

Put differently, these predicative relationships, such as the letter before the intervention, ground and construct the normative sequence. In the gender clinic, many enactments of gender are unimportant to medicine's sequence – legal name change, how one cuts one's hair, wearing a binder – but the predicative relationship of enactments bring a sequence into being.

Holding cis and trans patients against one another, it is clear that the letter of support enacts transness because there is doubt. Yet the letter also enacts transness in the face of doubt. These two readings of the letter's enactment are not mutually exclusive. Transness is enacted in the letter by a patient, a psychotherapist, and the clinician who requires the letter. This is done because of the high epistemological stakes of gender in societal systems such as biomedicine, the law, the household, etc. (Butler 1990; Kessler 1990; Spade 2006). Transness is held as an epistemological challenge to the gender binary, and thus is doubted and regulated (Plemons 2010; Spade 2006). However, the gender clinic also requires a letter of support in the face of this doubt. The endocrinologist and clinical social worker are invested in and committed to the trans community. In interviewing the clinical social worker, she stresses that she knows "that medicine has not always been kind to that entire population, not just trans, but to LGBT+ together... [W]ith such a marginalized population, I could understand how hard it would be to gain their trust. And trust was really important to us, because once you gain their trust you don't want to fail them... especially with minors, which is a very new, very controversial concept and treatment." Thus, by requiring a letter of support and following the international standards of care, the clinic is ensuring that medical care can be provided to these trans children, despite societal doubts about their existence. Doubt engenders predication, but an insistence on predication keeps the clinic open.

Other relations of predication beyond the letter of support construct a normative sequence within the gender clinic. For example, a patient must begin puberty before they can receive blockers.

It's immediately clear that Eric is shy when I follow the endocrinologist into her first consult of her afternoon clinic. Eric slouches in his chair, answering questions with a deep shrug so that his shoulders nearly reach the pink tips to his short brown hair. Eric's mother reports to the doctor that Eric started feeling pain in one of his nipples, so they went to their family doctor who confirmed breast development was beginning.

"After the pediatrician said it was the beginning of puberty, we made the appointment with you." Eric's mom says. "You told us to come if we saw signs of puberty."
"How long ago did this start, Eric?" the endocrinologist asks. Eric shrugs, but his mom answers, "Two months."
"Do you want to stop breast development?" the doctor asks. Again, Eric shrugs.
"Honey, you have to voice up and let us know what you want," Eric's mom tells him.
"I don't want to do anything you don't want to do," the doctor says, scrubbing in for the physical exam. "Do you want to have your breasts continue to grow?" the doctor finally asks pointe blanc.
"No, I don't want my breasts to continue growing," Eric says.
After the physical exam in which the endocrinologist confirms that breast development – female puberty – has begun, she tells Eric and his mom, "Well if we don't want the breast development to proceed, with blockers we have a plan. We can do injections, patch, or we can do the implant."
"Remember that implant we saw at our last visit?" Eric's Mom asks him. He nods a yes, and says he'd rather do the implant than the shots.
After our goodbyes, the doctor and I return to the workroom where she orders labs for Eric and a referral for the implant to be put in. She begins dictating her notes with, "Patient is tanner 2, so we can begin puberty suppression." [5]

For Eric breast development, a bodily enactment of female, must predicate a medical intervention to stop such bodily enactments. The gender clinic requires that all patients who receive blockers begin mis-gendered puberty. This is why they inform patients (and their caregivers) to look for the first sign of puberty and then schedule an appointment.

Like the letter of support from the psychotherapist, the gender clinic establishes this predicative relationship to dispel doubt. The common challenge to pediatric gender clinics by critics is that children and adolescents are not mature enough to make informed decisions about procedures and interventions that have permanent consequences, which hormone treatment does. Consequently, the endocrinologist references 'cognition' as the basis for requiring patients to begin a mis-gendered puberty before they can begin blockers. This 'cognition' signifies a patient is mature enough to offer 'assent' to

---

5   Tanner stages are stages of puberty on a scale of one to five, with one being pre-pubertal, and five being full pubertal maturity (Marshall and Tanner 1969; 1970). Of note, puberty blockers must be administered before tanner stage three, and early bodily changes in puberty can recede if blockers are administered early in puberty.

blockers (the parent must still offer 'consent') and has rejected their natal sexed puberty. The doctor explains that there is no physiological necessity to wait for puberty to begin; rather, the mis-gendered puberty is a tool that confirms the patient's rejection of a past gender and desire for a gender transition. In short, puberty becomes a litmus test. Thus, though Eric may have wanted to begin blockers at previous visits, he was told that he had to wait until he (or his mom) saw the first signs of female puberty.

Transness comes into being in this predicative relation between mis-gendered puberty and blockers. The bodily enactment of female gender as breast tissue, and the enactment of blockers as the absence of gender are practices that cross Eric's body. As I argued previously, a reality of transness is enacted as these practices are held in conflict. Moreover, we see a 'transition' in their sequencing. Eric transitions *from* female *to* male when these enactments – past, mis-gendered enactments; his current enactments of gender; and future, ideal enactments – are done in sequence. Predicative relationships establish this normative sequence: a letter of support always predicates medical intervention; a mis-gendered puberty always predicates blockers.

Khalif, the youngest trans- patient I meet in the clinic, is not considered for blockers during his visit because he has not started puberty. Logan must obtain a letter of support before the endocrinologist will prescribe him hormones. Eric begins blockers only now that he has had some breast tissue growth. All of these patients will have to wait until they are sixteen years old to begin HRT, and, per standards of care, will need a second letter of support to undergo any surgical procedures when they are eighteen or older. To participate in the gender clinic's intervention, Khalif, Logan, and Eric must fall into the normative sequence established by predicative relationships between ontologies of gender.

While predication can be thought of as a coordination of multiple realities of gender, sometimes various enactments conflict. One enactment may obstruct one specific reality of gender or transness from being enacted, or one reality may take preference in certain spaces, obstructing another from view.

An example of one of the simplest instances of obstruction in the clinic occurs, when a patient has their blood drawn to test hormone levels—testosterone and estrogen, most importantly. Vials of blood are taken to a lab, a space outside of the consultation and work rooms of the clinic, where they are analyzed. The vials of blood do not return to the clinic; instead, concentrations of hormones are sent back as test results. When looking at these hormone levels on her computer screen (all of the tests are reported digitally in the electronic medical health record), the doctor does not see a patient's social transition. Haircuts and clothing, pronouns and binders do not appear in the blood test. Blood test results – gender as hormone concentrations – obstruct many other enactments of gender from view.

Now, of course, this can be done in reverse and across many other gender-enactments. The clinical social worker's intake packet tells nothing of a patient's chromosomes. Gender enacted as hormone levels are obscured from a psychotherapist's letter. There are also times in which certain enactments of gender don't simply obstruct another enactment from view, but rather preclude other enactments of gender from coming into being. Such obstruction can be leveraged for clinical purposes – for example, blockers occlude an unwanted pubertal path – but it can also cause violence. Lily offers an example of this:

> I meet Lily, a cheery middle schooler, at their first appointment at the gender clinic. They have a soft-spoken nature and cross their legs tightly when sitting on the exam table. Lily identifies as gender fluid and uses they/them/theirs pronouns; however, they tell the doctor they would like to "transition to female" and use she/her/hers pronouns in the future. This desire is why they are at the clinic, now.
>
> The doctor is the first to see Lily. The consult begins with the doctor asking Lily about her gender identity and why she has come to the clinic. She then asks questions that are couched both as ways to build rapport and gain an understanding of the Lily's life and gender expression outside the clinic. "How is school?" the doctor asks Lily.
>
> "Um... Alright, I guess. I've got some friends, but I get teased," Lily says sitting on top of the exam table.
>
> "The school isn't great," Lily's mom adds from her spot sitting on a chair in the corner. "They're not very supportive. Lily can't use the bathroom she would like, and the teachers and administration don't do enough to stop the bullying. The teachers still call Lily by their male name and don't use the right pronouns."
>
> "And are you out at school?" the doctor asks.
>
> "No. We talked to the school about using my name and pronouns, but they weren't supportive," Lily responds.
>
> "Lily and I have talked about this and we decided it will be best for them to wait to transition and come-out at school until they go to high school," Lily's mom says.
>
> "And how do you feel about that, Lily?" the doctor asks, "Is that ok for you?"
>
> "Mmm-yeah," Lily answers.
>
> The doctor turns from Lily for a moment to write this in her notes on the computer. The doctor then asks, "And how are things at home?"

Lily and their mom explain that Lily's father is "not on board". That he thinks Lily's trans identity will "turn Lily's younger sister trans, too." That he won't use Lily's chosen name, or the gender-neutral nickname the family came up with. Lily's mother is supportive: she's brought Lily to the clinic and always uses Lily's pronouns and chosen name, but she feels torn between her husband and her child.

When we leave the consultation room and return to the workroom, the doctor briefs the clinical social worker on the consult. She reports Lily's name and pronouns, goes over some of their medical history and the medical exam – that they have started puberty, but are still in the early stages, so blockers will still be effective – and recounts Lily's experience at home and at school. The doctor ends by saying, "They're a good candidate [for treatment], except for their dad."

Here, Lily's father linguistically enacts maleness onto Lily by continuing to use a male name and male pronouns when speaking about them. By not recognizing Lily's chosen name and pronouns, Lily's father is blocking, obstructing, a relational linguistic enactment of Lily's gender fluidity (and femininity) from coming into being. Furthermore, because of Lily's father's legal power over them, his use of male pronouns and rejection of Lily's gender identity can obstruct other realities of gender. This is why we hear the doctor say, "They're a good candidate except for their dad". Lily's father's linguistic enactments of maleness could cross Lily's body and obstruct the sequence of gender affirming enactments the gender clinic provides for its patients. In fact, it is possible that if Lily cannot access gender-affirming care, Lily may miss the window to begin puberty blockers (before tanner stage 2) and their body will further corporally enact maleness in permanent ways – bone development, voice deepening, facial hair – as puberty progresses. Thus, Lily's father's use of former pronouns and names upholds its own sequence, one antithetical to Lily's gender identity, but one that, because it is imbued with power, has the ability to obstruct the realities of their gender Lily would like to enact.

Luckily for Lily, only one parent is required to provide consent for blockers. In turn, Lily is given a prescription for blockers and told to return in four months to monitor their hormone levels. Yet if Lily had been older and seeking HRT, the gender clinic would be more hesitant to prescribe HRT. In Lily's case, the benefit of blockers is that they have no positive effects: they will only stop puberty from beginning, rather than provide the 'feminizing effects' estrogen does. However, because of Lily's father's rejection of their gender identity, because of his enacting male with "he", Lily could be put in danger – harassed or kicked out of their house by their father – by taking estrogen and beginning a positive, medical transition. The gender clinic would not start Lily on HRT until they had Lily's father's consent and it was safe for Lily to begin a medical transition.[6] In this case, we see a masculine enactment, "he", obstructing enactments of femininity and gender fluidity – such as estrogen concentrations in Lily's blood, breast development, and fat redistribution – from coming into being.

Lily also experiences mis-gendering at school. Enacting gender as names and pronouns requires at least two actors: in this case, Lily and a teacher or the school administration. In refusing to participate in the linguistic enactments of Lily's gender as gender fluid or female, the school forecloses relational and social realities of gender fluid or female from being enacted, instead perpetuating Lily's enactment as male. "He" again obstructs gender fluidity and femininity enacted as "Lily" from coming into being.

Yet a medical transition would not necessarily be obstructed by the school's mis-gendering enactments. The school does not have the same power over Lily as their father does. In fact, while the gender clinic would never begin a medical transition if it thought doing so would put the patient in harm's way, the gender clinic applies its normative sequence so as to alleviate the violence a patient receives from society. The clinical social worker explains to me that the gender clinic is treating an incongruence between the patient's "body not matching their inside," but also "society saying that you're not normal." That is, the clinic understands that in some social spaces – such as schools – a dissonance between gender enactments, for instance a female name and pronouns and male skeletal shape and hair distribution, can place a child or adolescent at risk of violence.[7] Consequently, the gender clinic provides care that allows patients to bring bodily enactments of gender into reality under a logic that aligning the body with one's gender identity and expression decreases one's risk of violence.

The comparison of the possible violence of Lily's family and Lily's school leads to a critical point. The normative sequence of the gender clinic imagines a normative trans- subject, but it also expresses an assumption about where violence occurs: in society; that is, schools, extra-curricular activities,

---

6   In such cases, the clinic, especially the clinical social worker, would work with the family until it was safe for Lily to begin hormones.

7   While there are numerous high-profile cases of such violence, the recent work of Gayle Salamon, *The Life and Death of Latisha King: A Critical Phenomenology of Transphobia* (2018), offers in-depth scholarly coverage of one such case.

public spaces. However, Lily demonstrates that while violence can be societal, it is also intimate. That is, violence can come from one's own family. This is a violence that the normative sequence of the gender clinic cannot account for. It is an intimate violence of obstruction that causes a break, a pause, a block, a rupture in a child or adolescent's transition. The irony of the gender clinic's sequence is that a parent's support is necessary for a patient to enter the space of the clinic and for the sequence to even begin. Though the gender clinic aims to alleviate violence against trans youth, its normative sequence precludes those most at risk of violence – trans children with unaccepting parents – from accessing its services. In the context of trans youth suicide, this irony of the gender clinic's intervention assumes a morbid nature.

Lily's story is accordingly unlike that of the majority of patients in the clinic. Most have two supportive parents: an (at least mostly) accepting relationship between parent and child is what brings the patient to the gender clinic in the first place. Minors cannot make doctor's appointments without their parent's support, nor can they give consent.[8] Put plainly, children with unaccepting parents are rarely seen in the gender clinic. Thus, Lily's case reveals the original predicative relation of the gender clinic: the cooperation of parent and child must predicate the initiation of the gender clinic's sequence. Lily allows us to see the genesis and the morbid irony of the gender clinic's sequence.

While the relationship of obstruction exhibits how enactments can (permanently) forestall both sequences and other enactments from coming into existence or being seen, the relationship of justification has a converse effect. Justifying relationships accelerate the normative sequence of the clinic.

Beginning HRT is the point where justification most prominently comes into play because HRT is a point of predication (16 and having a letter of support) that has some 'wiggle room'. Most of the predicative relationships within the gender clinic follow strict rules: a patient *must* have a letter of support to begin hormone therapy or blockers; patients *must* have a second letter of support, have had twelve months of hormone therapy, and have lived twelve months openly as their gender identity before they can have gender affirmative surgeries (Coleman et al. 2012). However, the requirement that patients be at least sixteen years old before they are allowed to begin a hormone therapy

---

8   A court order can supersede a parent's lack of consent. This happens in the clinic when the care team believes the patient is at risk of suicide if the patient does not receive medical assistance with their transition.

has variability. New 2017 Endocrine Society practice guidelines state, "there may be compelling reasons to initiate sex hormone treatment prior to the age of 16 years in some adolescents with GD [Gender Dysphoria]/gender incongruence" (Hembree et al. 2017). While the standards offer thirteen and a half to fourteen years old as an earliest age to begin "sex hormone treatment," the pediatric gender clinic I study takes a more conservative approach, allowing some patients to begin receiving HRT at fifteen years of age.

In these cases, some outside factor, some other enactment of gender, allows the patient to enact gender as hormone levels and all of its consequent corporeal enactments sooner. Hormones produce some permanent changes. Consequently, the gender clinic follows the *Endocrine Society* guidelines, which state patients should only receive hormone treatment before they are sixteen years old if they have "sufficient mental capacity to give informed consent" (Hembree et al. 2017:3870). The logic of accelerating care, though, does not track in the gender clinic solely as a "mental capacity to give informed consent." Rather, the doctor might prescribe hormones when a patient is fifteen if she and the clinical social worker also "know" the patient is trans. This relation is labeled justification because the patient or an outside event must validate this "knowing" against any potential doubt in the patient's trans identity. That is, the patient must prove that they will not, as the social worker tells me, "desist from their cross-gender identification," in order to justify beginning hormone therapy early. In the current political climate[9] that surrounds trans children, desisting could lead to negative publicity for the gender clinic, causing it to limit its activity or even shut down. As such, "knowing" becomes a necessary justification for acceleration, in order that the clinic may continue to provide care for trans children and adolescents into the future.

Most of the clinical encounters that I observe in which "knowing" cumulates in beginning hormone therapy at age 15 rather than 16 are characterized by joy from the patients. They beam, ecstatic that a dream of theirs is

---

9   Political attacks on trans youth have taken on a chimeric form in the United States. Many of these laws, either proposed or ratified, have challenged trans children and adolescents' existence within public spaces. For instance, multiple states have challenged trans young people's use of bathrooms that align with their gender identity (Kralik 2019) and stopped trans youth from competing on school sports teams (GLSEN 2019). In 2020, a wave of states proposed laws against gender affirmative care for trans children and adolescents (Lam 2020). Being denied access to bathrooms associated with their gender identity and gender-appropriate college housing has been associated with increased suicidality (Seelman 2016).

coming true, and that a year of waiting has disappeared. Yet the calculus of "knowing" is never outright described. It appears often in the clinic, but its logic is left amorphous. The doctor tells Kalif's mother that hormone replacement therapy normally starts at 16 years old at the earliest, but if "we *know* the child is trans, we can start hormones earlier" (emphasis mine). She tells another patient and her mother, "We begin patients on gender affirming therapy [HRT] at 16, but it's possible to begin estrogen before 16 when we really *know*" (emphasis mine). There is no rubric or scale by which the clinic attempts to measure the transness of its patients. In fact, numerous times, the doctor and the clinical social worker stress to me—and also demonstrate with their actions—that they do not have an agenda for what a transition should look like, where it should end, or how a patient should identify and express themselves. Instead, it appears "knowing" is grounded in a trust between the patient and the gender clinic. Though not explicitly stated, this trust is founded upon compliance and consensus. Compliance insofar as the patient must be a 'good patient', one who makes their appointments, has their letter of recommendation, goes to therapy, etc.[10] And consensus between actors – therapists, parents, the social worker, the doctor – that the patient understands the risks and benefits of hormone therapy and does not doubt their gender identity. When all of the parties agree, when the gender clinic "knows" the patient is trans, the sequence can be accelerated so HRT can begin.

One patient, June, is told she can begin HRT when her father informs the doctor that June competes in trampoline gymnastics, and she may be qualify-

---

10   Racial and ethnic differences in compliance have been shown for various treatments, but it is unclear "whether they are due to differences in the way patients are treated or advised, in the cultural background of each patient, or in other factors" (Bulatao and Anderson 2004). While I did not observe any racial bias in the gender clinic, people of color are known to experience bias within medical settings that often leads to worse "patient–provider interactions, treatment decisions, treatment adherence, and patient health outcomes" (Hall et al. 2015). We also know that racial bias leads to less treatment and acknowledgement of people of color's pain as compared to white patients (Meghani, Byun and Gallagher 2012; Hoffman et al. 2016). Knowing that people of color may need to 'prove' their needs in medical spaces, it is possible people of color felt they had to especially prove their transness in order to receive medical care at the pediatric gender clinic. While I did not observe patients of color attempt to 'prove' their transness more than white patients, in my interviews and clinical interactions, many patients did express an (later admittedly unrealized) expectation to prove their gender identity and/or their worthiness for trans healthcare before entering the pediatric gender clinic.

ing for the national championships this year. She needs to meet the Olympic standards for testosterone levels to be able to compete in the women's category. This enactment of June's gender, competing in the women's category, justifies beginning estrogen therapy before June is 16 years old. "Knowing" is present in June's clinical visit, though the word is never said. She is one of the care team's favorite patients (they tell me so), and the care team views her as a compliant patient. If the consensus of June's gender from this outside actor is founded on certain hormone levels, and the gender clinic 'knows' June as trans, then extending this 'knowledge' justifies beginning estrogen therapy early.

Further evidence of "knowing" as justification for beginning HRT therapy early can be found in the contrapositive cases: when the doctor and social worker feel a patient should not begin hormone therapy early. There are not many patients the care team feels, who must wait until they are 16 to begin HRT, but Aaron offers an example of one:

> I meet Aaron when I observed his clinical visit; however, I am not able to observe his time with the clinical social worker. When the care team reconvenes in the workroom, the clinical social worker asks in regard to Aaron, "Taking testosterone increases your risk of stroke, right? Both his father and his grandfather died young because of stroke. So, I asked him, 'How are you going to deal with that risk?' Aaron said he would eat healthy and exercise, but then I asked him, 'Didn't your dad also eat healthy and exercise?'"
>
> By the end of their discussion, both the doctor and the clinical social worker agree that Aaron "is a patient we should really wait until 16 with. He may not have the maturity to understand the risk of taking these hormones and we need to wait until he understands the risks more."
>
> A training clinical social worker then asks the clinical social worker, "Is the patient immature?"
>
> The clinical social worker replies, "Aaron isn't immature for a natal male, but he is immature for a natal female."

All of the staff of the gender clinic address Aaron by his male name and use he/him/his pronouns – the ones he told them he uses. They accept Aaron as trans and don't visibly doubt his identity. At the same time, the doctor and the clinical social worker are not convinced Aaron "gets the risk of" and can provide informed consent for the medical intervention he wishes the undergo. 'Maturity' is obstructing an acceleration of the clinic's normative sequence.

The clinical social worker also states that at Aaron's age, natal females should be mature, whereas natal males are immature. In a sense, Aaron's immaturity should enact male, then. He is meeting medicine's epistemological understanding of maturity and development for the male sex. However, the conclusion the gender clinic reaches is because Aaron's assigned sex at birth is female, and because he is not mature when a female should be mature, he is developmentally behind and cannot give consent. While the care team would never explicitly doubt Aaron's gender identity, in employing Aaron's natal sex to establish his maturity, the clinical social worker and doctor continue to enact femaleness in Aaron. This enactment of female breaks a potential consensus of actors enacting maleness with Aaron. There is still some doubt with female still being done, still present. Therefore, through the language of maturity and informed consent, the gender clinic does not fully 'know' Aaron is trans, and he cannot accelerate his transition.

In sum, Aaron's and June's stories demonstrate that the relationship of justification accelerates the normative sequence of the clinic. This acceleration is unobtainable to Aaron and other patients, for whom a consensus of 'knowing' cannot be reached, or for those who are considered non-compliant patients. Acceleration takes advantage of the changing recommendations of when to begin hormone therapy, but it must be justified because the clinic is betting against patients "desisting from their cross-gender identification." In short, gender enacted as the clinic 'knowing' a patient's gender identity justifies accelerating the normative sequence and prescribing HRT before the age of sixteen.

Conclusion

In this chapter, I have explored the ontology of gender and transness within a United States pediatric care clinic and employed this exploration to examine the temporal sequence of gender transitions. While engaging ethnographic data, I outlined the ways in which Mol's theory of "ontology as practice" can be applied to a pediatric gender clinic. Realities of gender come into being through practices, and trans ontologies appear in the conflict of gender ontologies, often through temporal rupture. Building on this, I explored through vignettes how predicative relationships between enactments construct the normative sequence of transition within the gender clinic, and how obstructive and justifying relationships slow, halt or accelerate this normative sequence.

Within the framework of relationships between enactments I elucidate the original predicate of the pediatric gender clinic: that the patients of the gender clinic must have their parents' support to access its resources—an assumption of the location of violence, and in turn, a morbid irony. The gender clinic aims to mitigate violence against trans youth by providing affirming medical care; however, this original predicate forecloses access to the gender clinic's resources to those trans children experiencing the most intimate of violence. Said differently, the normative sequence cannot account for the intimate violence that trans youth without supportive parents experience by being precluded from accessing the gender clinic's resources.

Mol closes her book, *The Body Multiple* (2002), by asking "What reality should we live with?" (Mol 2002:165). While not directly taking this question on, this chapter allows us to see that the gender clinic's normative timeline has a utilitarian value, but also strands in relation to structural and intimate violence as a predicate to entering the clinic's doors. Thinking about the open-ended relationship of the term 'trans', how might the gender clinic build coalitions of care with actors beyond the hospital walls to reach and support those trans youth precluded from its care (Stryker, Currah and Moore 2008)? And how might the clinic make space for trans youth enacting realities not accounted for within its normative sequence? Trans youth both within and outside the normative timeline of care are navigating shifting landscapes of predication, obstruction, and acceleration. With its seat within biomedicine, the pediatric gender clinic has the power to shape what realities they and we should live with.

References

Becerra-Culqui, T.A.; Lui, Y.; Nash, R.; Cromwell, L.; Flanders, W.D.; Getahun, D.; Giammattei, S.V.; Hunkeler, E.M.; Lash, T.L.; Millman, A.; Quinn, V.P.; Robinson, B.; Roblin, D.; Sanberg, D.E.; Silverberg, M.J.; Tangpricha, V. and Goodman, M. (2018): Mental Health of Transgender and Gender Nonconforming Youth Compared With Their Peers. Pediatrics. In: American Academy of Pediatrics, 141(5), p. e20173845.

Benjamin, H. (1954): Transsexualism and Transvestism as Psychosomatic and Somatopsychic Syndromes. In: American Journal of Psychotherapy, 8(2), pp. 219–230.

Berlant, L. (2011): Cruel Optimism. Durham: Duke University Press.

Bulatao, R.A. and Anderson, N.B. (Eds) (2004): Understanding Racial and Ethnic Differences in Health in Late Life: A Research Agenda. Washinton, DC: National Academies Press.

Butler, J. (1990): Gender Trouble and the Subversion of Identity. New York and London: Routledge.

Coleman, E.; Bockting, W.; Botzer, M. and Cohen-Kettenis, P.T. (2012): Standards of Care for the Health of Transsexual, Transgender, and Gender-Nonconforming People, Version 7. In: International Journal of Transgenderism, 13(4), pp. 165–232.

Freeman, E. (2010): Time Binds: Queer Temporalities, Queer Histories. Durham: Duke University Press.

Gay, Lesbian and Straight Education Network (GLSEN, 2019): Transgender Inclusion in High School Athletics [online]. Available at: https://www.glsen.org/sites/default/files/2019-10/GLSEN-Transgender-Inclusion-High-School-Athletics.pdf (Accessed: 04 December 2021).

Gill-Peterson, J. (2018): Histories of the Transgender Child. Minnesota: University of Minnesota Press.

Haas, A.P.; Rodgers, P.L. and Herman, J. (2014): Suicide Attempts among Transgender and Gender Non-Conforming Adults: Findings of the National Transgender Discrimination Survey. Los Angeles: The Williams Institute.

Hall, W.J.; Chapman, M.V.; Lee, K.M.; Merino, J.M.; Thomas, T.W.; Payne, B.K.; Eng, E.; Day, S.H. and Beasley, T.C. (2015): Implicit Racial/Ethnic Bias Among Health Care Professionals and Its Influence on Health Care Outcomes: A Systematic Review. In: American Journal of Public Health, 105(12), pp. 60-76.

Hembree, W.C.; Cohen-Kettenis, P.T.; Delemarre-van de Waal, H.A.; Gooren, L.J.; Meyer 3rd, W.J.; Spack, N.P.; Tangpricha, V.; Montori, V.M. and Endocrine Society (2009): Endocrine Treatment of Transsexual Persons: An Endocrine Society Clinical Practice Guideline. In: The Journal of Clinical Endocrinology and Metabolism, 94(9), pp. 3132–3154.

Hembree, W.C; Cohen-Kettenis P.T.; Gooren, L.; Hannema, S.E.; Meyer, W.J.; Murad, M.H.; Rosenthal, S.M.; Safer, J.D.; Tangpricha, V. and T'Sjoen, G.G. (2017): Endocrine Treatment of Gender-Dysphoric/Gender-Incongruent Persons: An Endocrine Society Clinical Practice Guideline. In: The Journal of Clinical Endocrinology and Metabolism, 102(11), pp. 3869–3903.

Hoffman, K.M.; Trawalter, S.; Axt, J.R. and Oliver, M.N. (2016): Racial Bias in Pain Assessment and Treatment Recommendations, and False Beliefs about Biological Differences between Blacks and Whites. In: Proceedings of the National Academy of Sciences of the United States of America, 113(16), pp. 4296–4301.

Kessler, S.J. (1990): The Medical Construction of Gender: Case Management of Intersexed Infants. In: Signs: Journal of Women in Culture and Society, 16(1), pp. 3–26.

Kralik, J. (2019): "Bathroom Bill" Legislative Tracking. In: NCSL, 24 October 2019 [online]. Available at: https://www.ncsl.org/research/education/-bathroom-bill-legislative-tracking635951130.aspx (Accessed: 04 December 2021).

Lam, K. (2020): National firestorm on horizon as states consider criminalizing transgender treatments for youths. In: USA Today, n.d. [online]. Available at: https://eu.usatoday.com/story/news/nation/2020/02/06/transgender-youth-transition-treatment-state-bills/4605054002/ (Accessed: 04 December 2021).

Latham, J.R. (2017): (Re) Making Sex: A Praxiography of the Gender Clinic. In: Feminist Theory, 18(2), pp. 177–204.

Marshall, W.A. and Tanner, J.M. (1969): Variations in the Pattern of Pubertal Changes in Girls. In: Archives of Disease in Childhood, 44(235), pp. 291-303.

Marshall, W.A. and Tanner, J.M. (1970): Variations in the Pattern of Pubertal Changes in Boys. In: Archives of Disease in Childhood, 45(239), pp. 13-23.

Meghani, S.H.; Byun, E. and Gallagher, R.M. (2012): Time to Take Stock: A Meta-Analysis and Systematic Review of Analgesic Treatment Disparities for Pain in the United States. In: Pain Medicine, 13(2), pp. 150–174.

Minnesota Department of Health (2019): 2019 Minnesota Student Survey Results Released [online]. Available at: https://www.health.state.mn.us/news/pressrel/2019/studentsurvey101719.html (Accessed: 04 December 2021).

Mol, A. (2002): The Body Multiple: Ontology in Medical Practice. Durham: Duke University Press.

Nock, M.K; Borges, G.; Bromet, E.J.; Cha, C.B.; Kessler, R.C. and Lee, S. (2008): Suicide and Suicidal Behavior. In: Epidemiologic Reviews, 30(1), pp. 133–154.

Salamon, G. (2018): The Life and Death of Latisha King: A Critical Phenomenology of Transphobia. New York: NYU Press.

Seelman, K.L. (2016): Transgender adults' access to college bathrooms and housing and the relationship to suicidality. In: Journal of Homosexuality, 63, (10), pp. 1378–1399.

Spade, D. (2006): Mutilating Gender. In: Whittle, S. and Stryker, S. (Eds.): The Transgender Studies Reader. New York: Taylor & Francis, pp. 315–332.

Spade, D. (2015): Normal Life: Administrative Violence. Critical Trans Politics, and the Limits of Law. Durham: Duke University Press.

Stockton, K.B. (2009): The Queer Child, or Growing Sideways in the Twentieth Century. Durham: Duke University Press.

Stryker, S.; Currah, P. and Jean Moore, L. (2008): Introduction: Trans-, Trans, or Transgender? In: WSQ: Women's Studies Quarterly, 36(3), pp. 11–22.

Whitbeck, L.; Welch Lazoritz, M.; Crawford, D. and Hautala, D. (Eds.) (2014): Street Outreach Program. Data Collection Project Executive Summary [online]. Available at: https://www.rhyttac.net/assets/docs/Research/rese arch%20-%20sop%20data%20collection%20project.pdf (Accessed: 04 December 2021).

The Parallel Process of Trans Mental Health Providers – The Strengths and Complexities of Working as a Trans Person in Mental Healthcare

Omer Elad

I have been part of the trans community for nearly two decades, and a social worker weaving in and out of working with trans people in professional capacities for a decade. The intersection of those identities presented a myriad of opportunities to reflect on my role and the complicated context of trans identities and social services, especially trans healthcare. Along the way, I stumbled on the concept of the parallel process, which I have found useful in this context. In this chapter, I apply the concept of parallel process in an extended reflection on my personal and professional experience as a trans person working in the mental health system.

Parallel process is defined as "a treatment impasse that occurs when similar emotional difficulties emerge simultaneously in supervisory and treatment relationships" (Kahn 1979:520). This concept has fascinated me since the beginning of my social work career. As a graduate student, I was an assistant for research focused on the parallel processes that can occur when social workers are working within communities with whom they share a common identity-based experiences. I interviewed gay social work students working in LGBTQ centers, black social work students working in predominantly black neighborhoods of Boston, and in similar situations. The experiences reported to me were complex and nuanced. In my own career as a person who holds multiple identities outside of the hegemony, I have found myself frequently grappling with experiences of parallel process. I've witnessed their multidimensional impact on therapeutic relationships with clients and with supervisors alike. Most illuminating was exploring my own trans and non-binary identities while working with trans and non-binary clients or service recipients. Drawing on my own experiences, as well as existing research, I will draw some conclusions about the emotional difficulties that emerge in this context, as well as the joyous successes that can significantly remove barriers and improve care.

I am an unlicensed social worker working in community mental health and housing access in the West Coast of North America. I am a white immigrant, a person with a disability, and I am trans non-binary and queer. My career has taken place in community mental health settings that are not deliberately trans-affirming. In this acknowledgment, I seek to locate my positionality, a concept which "directly incorporates ideas of power and privileges and seeks to describe researcher identity in terms of insider-outsider perspective, based on the researchers' relationship to the specific research setting and community" (Muhammad et al. 2015:4). While this chapter is not significantly research-based, those identities and others inform and shape my analysis. Additionally, language and culture are constantly evolving to better include and reflect dynamic concepts. I use the overall term 'trans' to include trans, gender non-conforming and non-binary identities. This helps to simplify my discussion but is by no means intended to limit further explorations of these categories.

The last two decades brought an increasing need for trans-specific services as well as increased visibility of mental health providers who are trans (Lurie 2014). However, in part due to discrimination and systemic barriers to education, wealth, and professional development (James et al. 2016) trans providers in the US are rare. Each is often the sole or one of the few providers with trans competency within a local system of care. As Shuster (2016: 329) puts it, "despite insightful research on the experience of trans people in workplace organizations and everyday life [...] there are still few studies on trans medicine, particularly from the providers' perspective." Meanwhile, trans therapists such as Hansbury (2011:212) report: "because I am publicly 'out', trans patients routinely come to me specifically seeking a trans therapist. In their own words and actions, they tell me they are looking for an experience of twinship and mirroring." The literature on the subject of trans mental health providers working with trans clients is limited in its scope. For this essay, I rely heavily on few existing articles as well as unpublished thesis papers. I also draw on my experience as a trans mental health provider in community mental health settings in the US.

While the concept of parallel process specifically seeks to illuminate difficulties, I argue that it should be considered for its benefits as well. Everett et al. (2013) discuss the ethics of multiple relationships within queer, two-spirit[1], and/or trans communities in a similar vein, arguing that while these relationships are perceived as negative and potentially harmful in traditional ethical analysis, they may also have potential benefits. Here, I will explore some ways in which the trans-transference (Lurie 2014) and the trans-trans dyad (Hansbury 2011; Lurie 2014) impact the providers and the therapeutic relationships.

In an attempt to embrace the complexity of relationality, I seek to look beyond the binary labelling of experiences as "negative" or "positive". Borrowing from Buddhist concepts as well as behavioral neuroscience (Dolcos and Cabeza 2002), I choose to explore this topic using the lens of "pleasant" and "unpleasant". These concepts move away from a black and white thinking (something is either good or bad, right or wrong). It may offer a connection between the logical experience (interpreting our experience through morals, values, and past) with the somatic one (how does it feel in our body? How does it feel in our senses?).

It is 2014 and I start looking for a therapist for the first time since my teenage years. I am a medically-transitioned non-binary person and a mental health provider myself, already have navigated the hoops of medical care for many years, and as a result, I minimize my interactions with the medical system as much as possible. My body and my identities put me at risk of not receiving the care that I need. Often, therapists would focus on trans identities as focal to treatment due to their own biases. Other times, doctors in various disciplines may fail to treat trans people in emergency situations and primary care alike, treating trans bodies as foreign, sometimes as inhuman. It is a common saying in the community to joke about the "trans broken arm syndrome", phenomena in which doctors blame everything (including a broken arm) on the patient's trans identity, neglecting their care. I just separated from my spouse, alone in a country that is thousands of miles away from home, and like many of my peers, I want to do some self-work. I start inquiring. I type in 'transgender' and 'therapist' and 'sliding scale', I seek recommendations in forums and websites: 'looking for a trans-competent therapist'. Living in a big urban city on the West Coast of the United States, I am privileged to have access to many therapists, who claim a competency, but I am still unsure what it means for them, and so what it would mean for me. Some therapists who share my identities are also my peers, so not accessible

---

1   See Glossary at the beginning of this book.

to me as a client. I leave many tabs open in my browser, unsure how to proceed, and eventually take a deep breath and choose the one with an image
in which the therapist looks kind.

In our introductory meeting, I tell her about my deep fear of being sensa-
tionalized, I tell her who I am, a laundry list of identities, just a beginning,
and ask about who she is. I need to know. She is queer, she confirms, and
partnered with a trans person, too. I feel my shoulders relaxing, my breath
is easier. Ok, I tell myself, perhaps we have something to work with here.

While my therapist is not a trans person herself, her self-disclosure and
visibility removed a significant barrier in my access to competent services.
Visibility and self-disclosure are specifically highlighted in research as a
pleasant part of the parallel process of trans mental health providers and a
factor in the ability to provide affirming and competent services (Lurie 2014;
Karnoski 2017). Lurie (2014) discusses the idea of modeling vulnerability
("bringing more of me into the room," 2014:48) as a therapeutic intervention,
in which clients are able to witness and hold space for their therapist, and
subsequently practice vulnerability and compassion as skills for their own
lives. It has been my own experience that disclosure of trans status to trans
clients often leads to increased trust, openness and relationship building.
Moreover, trans providers have noted challenges in getting their own needs
met because of their role and the potential for crossover or conflict. Some
examples are accessing support groups, therapy, trans-affirming care, trans-
competent supervision, or attending community events and engagement
(Everett et al. 2013; Lurie 2014). This challenge has the potential to be unpleasant and lead to providers having a smaller life than before they entered
the trans-trans dyad. This dynamic puts them at risk of isolation, lessened
social support, and burn out. Shamai (2003:545) notes, "because helping professionals are themselves exposed to the political violence and uncertainty,
their personal experience of it may affect their professional performance
and result in feeling overwhelmed and burned out". As trans mental health
providers largely live in the same political climate which impacts their clients,
it is crucial to explore and seek to understand the nuanced way in which it
may show up in the therapeutic relationship and the parallel process.

Hansbury (2011:210) therefore asks, "with few examples against which to
compare myself, I am often left to wonder: Does the transgender analyst
work differently from the cisgender analyst? Are the issues experienced by
trans patients different from those those cis patients struggle with?" While

answers may differ, it is worth noting that culturally competent care must include those who are impacted by these issues. These people should not only be receiving services but also leading the implementation of care. Because of the unique cultural and sociopolitical aspect of trans healthcare worldwide, in which trans communities are simultaneously politicized as identities and medicalized as a measure of control, trans people are often dependent on providers. Mental health providers play a significant role as they are often required to 'assess' trans people before they are granted access to many forms of medical and social transition. Thus, trans mental health providers are often engaged in political activism. They lead transformations of workplaces and workplace ethics, and often occupy the position of role model due to their trans identity. While many find "purpose, meaning, and connection through [...] activist histories" (Lurie 2014: 61), this political context adds additional layers to their therapeutic relationships.

I graduate with my Masters of Social Work and start working as a social worker, providing therapy, case management and mental health support in the community. I get swept into the field of homelessness and mental health and decide not to work in LGBTQ-specific organizations. 'We are everywhere', I say. And we are. As I am largely out at my workplaces, trans people are typically referred to me wherever I work. I am cis-passing and have the privilege (or burden) of choosing self-disclosure, as I find fit and so I begin to navigate self-disclosure and its relation to the construction of my professional identity. I particularly love witnessing the shift in my clients when I disclose. Often it is apparent by the relaxation of their shoulders that they find more ease with the knowledge of my identity. I cannot claim neutrality. I feel a special kind of joy when I get my trans clients housed, when they make it to an appointment, when I can advocate with and for them, when they access trans-affirming services. I feel a certain kind of sorrow when they drop off treatment, when I cannot find them in the shelter or their tent – when barriers are too enormous to scale. I also start organizing in the local trans community, making relationships even more complex. As my activist network grows, I at times refer people to services through social media engagement. Knowing that I have the capacity to support community members in accessing services even in a hostile environment means a lot to me, but I am worried about what my co-workers and supervisors may say about my professional integrity.

Trans mental health workers walk a fine line within little-charted territory. We often become experts on providing trans-competent care (Everett et al. 2013; Lurie 2014), relying on our professional capacity, our activism, our own identities, and our own communities. At the same time, we engage with self-surveillance (Everett et al. 2013), are impacted by microaggressions in our workplaces (Nadal et al. 2014), and by de-professionalization or fear of it (Everett et al. 2013). Many of us can feel trapped at times and not recognized for expertise that is unrelated to trans issues (Lurie 2014). Beyond microaggression, providers often experience harm, discrimination, and trauma in their own work environment, which puts an additional burden on them as staff, risking unpleasant experiences of burn out and cycles of trauma when working with trans clients who navigate similar experiences. The pressure to be 'professional' is rooted in the dominant culture, in this case cis- and heteronormative culture[2]. It is essential to seek ways to challenge that and to address the parallel process in which providers and clients are harmed in parallel to their establishing of a therapeutic relationship.

Although trans clients often seek mirroring (Hansbury 2011), it is false to assume sameness in the trans-trans dyad. If we assume sameness of the therapist and clients solely because of their trans identities, we ignore the fact that power dynamics are inherent to the therapeutic relationship. Additionally, intersectionality (Crenshaw 1991) plays a significant part in this differentiation of roles. Despite sharing the trans identity, there are many ways in which those identities can play out differently in people's lives. When I am a white transmasculine therapist who has had access to education and financial stability and I work with a black trans woman, who is homeless, our experiences are not mirroring each other. Moreover, providers may experience a parallel process which can include envy or jealousy of their clients (Lurie 2014:48), assimilation bias (having preconceived thoughts about a trans person should do or be), and simply not being a good match due to personality or professional mismatch.

As a social work intern, I intern in a community health clinic for marginalized youth and young adults in Boston, MA. I get a small caseload of clients, some of them are trans. Most of the staff in the mental health team is queer.

---

2   Queer and/or trans healthcare providers often need to look, dress, speak, and conduct themselves in accordance to unspoken (and at times spoken) rules, often needing to 'tone down' queerness/transness in order to gain respect, validity, professional development, promotions, etc. in their workplace.

There is a therapist who is trans. He tells me he stopped going to community events to maintain professional boundaries. I grapple with this question of where my personal identity ends and where the professional one begins. I am not sure. As part of my job, I provide 'Gender Assessment', a too-elaborated process that clients are required to undergo in order to access medical transition. I start writing letters that my clients need in order to access hormones, or surgeries. I tell them I am trans too, I try out self-disclosure and consider the ways my disclosure can be beneficial for my work with them, but I am not sure about what is best. I am angry that I need to write these letters, grateful that I can do it collaboratively and with as few barriers as I can.

Trans healthcare is steeped in the medical model and many trans people are dependent on medical and mental healthcare to get their healthcare needs met. A recent study (Gonzalez and Henning-Smith 2017:743; 726) found that "transgender and GNC [gender nonconforming] adults were more likely to be uninsured, to have no usual source of care, and to forgo needed medical care due to cost," and that "transgender and GNC adults may experience barriers to care for a variety of reasons, including discrimination and lack of awareness by providers in healthcare settings". This highlights a particularly interesting aspect of the parallel process that occurs when a trans mental health provider acts as a gatekeeper of a client's access to medical care. In Lurie's research (2014) and my own experience, this situation elicits a range of responses from the healthcare provider. Some sit in discomfort, some attempt to work collaboratively with the client to navigate the administrative hurdle they are facing, and some choose not to assume this role at all. Many contemporary trans mental health providers choose to use their position of power to relieve gatekeeping where possible and make the process easier for their clients. They may only meet the minimum requirements of the guidelines or find loopholes, they may write those letters with their clients and empower clients to use their own words, and some may risk scrutiny of co-workers and supervisors for doing so. Everett et al. (2013) in particular point at the scrutiny that results from supervisors who lack trans-specific knowledge, and trans providers' fear of job insecurity and the ensuing self-surveillance. In a recent study of trans and non-binary medical students, Dimant et al. (2019:215) found that "in many cases, individuals hid their identity due to fear of discrimination, substantiated by witnessing high levels of anti-TNB [trans non-binary] stigma and discrimination. Both medical school and residency curricula have not sufficiently included TNB health topics nor changed transphobic attitudes. Even attending physicians reported environments that continued to perpetuate stigma and discrimination." Although this research focused on medical students and physicians, it is fair to deduce that the medical world is not preparing or prepared to support trans people and their needs. As a result, trans mental health providers, who are both clients of and gatekeepers of trans healthcare, are asked to carry an incredibly complicated load in support of their clients and their communities.

What would it look like to practice as a trans mental health provider in a world that did not medicalize trans people? In a world where the power to determine someone's readiness for treatment was not put in the hand of the provider? How would that change the trans-trans dyad and trans-transference?

> At the same internship, I worked with a young trans person who also explored their multiple identities. We worked in therapy on various coping strategies and their transition-related goals. When they were ready to pursue surgery, I felt confident in my ability to write them a letter and support them. However, my supervisor was concerned about the intersection of their mental health diagnosis and was not fully supportive of moving forward with the letter. The case had to be moved 'up the channel' and reviewed by other clinicians. I had to employ more advocacy and support my client as we were both navigating barriers to their care. Eventually, the case was approved and my client was able to access their care.

This particular experience remained poignant for me over the years of my professional development and is reflected in the existing research. On the one hand, trans providers are viewed as having more experience and expertise than their cisgender coworkers and often supervisors (Lurie 2014), but on the other hand, they are also questioned and undermined for this expertise (Karnoski 2017).

> I apply to a supervisory position, my current position. The team I would supervise is part of my interviews and I tell them right away, I am trans, I am queer, this is who I am. I tell them my pronouns, too. I get the job. We learn together. We share this learning process with our clients. We grow. I work for a large agency in a progressive West Coast American city and I am shocked to see how much work is needed for the organization to become trans-competent—for both staff and clients. I enthusiastically throw myself into the work

and start a working committee, where we all volunteer our time and expertise to improve the organization. We write a handout, we fix, we correct, we advocate, we are angry, we are shut down, we get misgendered (every day), our recommendations are at times dismissed, the system is slow to change, and the re-traumatization is alive and burning. On the workgroup some of us are therapists, some of us are peers, some of us are administrators, some of us are trans, some of us are allies. Our monthly meetings become a place of solace, support and solidarity, a community.

Exploring the concept of parallel process in the trans-trans dyad brings up more questions than answers. A lot is left to be researched, explored and conceptualized. Baril (2015:68) boldly states "trans suffering cannot be reduced to internalized cisgenderist oppression", and I postulate that this is true for trans joy as well. The experience and skills trans mental health providers bring to the field cannot be understated. The burden of the parallel process, as well as the immense joy, are equally significant in the impact they have on the well-being of providers. The importance of culturally competent services has been established as important to mental healthcare (National Association of Social Workers 2015), yet some of the challenges remain to be explored. As this exploration continues, it is critical to consider the significance of mirroring and counter-mirroring, where the provider's identity is reflected in their clients and vice versa. This unique situation creating a space with the potential of solace, support, solidarity, and healing for both client and provider.

References

Baril, A. (2015): Transness as Debility: Rethinking Intersections between Trans and Disabled Embodiments. In: Feminist Review, 111(1), pp. 59–74.

Crenshaw, K. (1991): Mapping the Margins: Intersectionality, Identity Politics, and Violence Against Women of Color. In: Stanford Law Review, 43(6), pp. 1241-1299.

Dimant, O.E.; Cook, T.E.; Greene, R.E. and Radix, A.E. (2019): Experiences of Transgender and Gender Nonbinary Medical Students and Physicians. In: Transgender Health 4(1), pp. 209–216.

Dolcos, F. and Cabeza, R. (2002): Event-Related Potentials of Emotional Memory: Encoding Pleasant, Unpleasant, and Neutral Pictures. In: Cognitive, Affective, and Behavioral Neuroscience, 2(3), pp. 252-263.

Everett, B.J.; Macfarlane, D.A.; Reynolds, V.A. and Anderson, H. (2013): Not On Our Backs: Supporting Counsellors in Navigating the Ethics of Multiple Relationships Within Queer, Two Spirit, and/or Trans Communities. In: Canadian Journal of Counselling and Psychotherapy, 47(1), pp. 14-28.

Gonzales, G. and Henning-Smith, C. (2017): Barriers to Care Among Transgender and Gender Nonconforming Adults. In: The Milbank Quarterly, 95(4), pp. 726-748.

Hansbury, G. (2011): King Kong & Goldilocks: Imagining Transmasculinities through the Trans–Trans Dyad. In: Psychoanalytic Dialogues, 21, pp. 210-220.

James, S.; Herman, J.; Rankin, S.; Keisling, M.; Mottet, L. and Anafi, M. (2016): Executive Summary of the Report of the 2015 U.S. Transgender Survey. Washington D.C.: National Center for Transgender Equality.

Kahn, E.M. (1979): The Parallel Process in Social Work Treatment and Supervision. In: Social Casework: The Journal of Contemporary Social Work, 60(9), pp. 520-528.

Karoski, R. (2017): Experience of Healthcare Providers of Lesbian, Gay, Bisexual, and Transgender Foster Youth. Unpublished Master's thesis. Seattle: University of Washington.

Lurie, S. (2014): Exploring the Impacts of Disclosure for Transgender and Gender Non-Conforming Therapists. Unpublished Master's thesis. Northampton: Smith College.

Muhammad, M.; Wallerstein, N., Sussman, A.L.; Avila, M.; Belone, L. and Duran, B. (2015): Reflections on Researcher Identity and Power: The Impact of Positionality on Community Based Participatory Research (CBPR) Processes and Outcomes. In: Critical Sociology, 41(7-8), pp. 1045–1063.

Nadal, K.L.; Davidoff, K.C.; Davis, L.S. and Wong, Y. (2014): Emotional, Behavioral, and Cognitive Reactions to Microaggressions: Transgender Perspectives. Psychology of Sexual Orientation and Gender Diversity, 1(1), pp. 72-81.

National Association of Social Workers (2015): Standards and Indicators for Cultural Competence in Social Work Practice [online]. Available at: https://www.socialserviceworkforce.org/system/files/resource/files/Standards%20and%20Indicators%20for%20Cultural%20Competence%20in%20Social%20Work%20Practice.pdf (Accessed 31 January 2022).

Shamai, M. (2003): Using Social Constructionist Thinking in Training Social Workers Living and Working under Threat of Political Violence, In: Social Work, 48(4), pp. 545–555.

Shuster, S.M. (2016): Uncertain Expertise and the Limitations of Clinical Guidelines in Transgender Healthcare. In: Journal of Health and Social Behavior, 57(3), pp. 319–332.

Ganda ng Transpinays:
Narratives on Trans Health, Barriers to Care and Trans Sisterhood in the Philippines

Brenda Rodriguez Alegre

Transpinay is one of the more current terms to denote of the identities of trans women in the Philippines. The term was introduced by STRAP, The Society of Transsexual Women of the Philippines, which has been around since 2002. Being the first and oldest existing trans organization in the Philippines, STRAP members have collectively shaped narratives that structure the experience of transpinays; for example, in terms of life development, integration into society, obstacles and prejudices, and the meaning of transition. Although this term was not often used in the Philippines until the early 2000s, there has been an ongoing tradition of transpinay communities supporting steps toward physical transition. The use of hormones and silicone injections and optional surgical procedures are often learned from other transpinays, mostly in the trans pageantry and local beauty salons. Those salons predominantly employ transpinays and gay men.

The absence of a gender recognition law, same-sex union law, anti-discrimination law and apparent exclusion in reproductive health law among others, are some of the reasons why transpinays refrain from accessing formal healthcare. They rather consult with each other, especially concerning questions about transitioning.

The dominant catholic culture brought to the Philippines by missionaries during the Spanish colonial years contributed to the erasure of pre-colonial gender non-normative identities, such as the babaylans and the catalonans[1].

---

1   Babaylans and catalonans are among the pre-colonial identities normative to varying regions of the Philippines. They share some similarities with pre-colonial Hijars of South Asia or Berdache of North America.

Colonization sets the context for the barriers to integration faced by trans people in the Philippines today.

This chapter provides a narrative of transpinays and some experiences of transpinoys (Philippine trans men). It shows how they navigate a conservative, traditional and politically divided Christian society on their journey to openly live their authentic selves. This chapter also explores the barriers trans people experience when transitioning and when accessing healthcare.

Most of all, I aim to account for how transpinays (and some transpinoys) manage to remain vibrantly visible in a society that is, paradoxically, both tolerant and unaccepting. I argue that sorority and fraternity among trans people is key to survival and to finding themselves when they get lost in transition.

Introduction

Prior to colonization, there were a number of significant gender-variant identities in the Philippines (Alegre 2013:15ff). These identities are the babaylans, the catalonans and the asogs, among others, which existed across indigenous groups in different provinces of the Philippines.

Filipinos were animists or pagans long before Christianity was introduced (Alegre 2013:15ff; Brewer 1999:14ff; Johnson 1997:25ff). The aforementioned identities were treated with respect and veneration similar to the hijras of South Asia or berdache of North America (Nanda 1998:xix; Roscoe 2016:9ff.). Their roles in our early society were like shamans or high priests, even community leaders. Since the Spanish colonization, those early identities were repressed and only preserved through oral history (Brewer 1999:14ff).

The Philippines has become a predominantly catholic country, yet it appears to be relatively tolerant towards LGBTIQ people (PEW Research Centre 2013). In current media and pop culture, LGBTIQ people are visible. One of the most renowned celebrities and entertainers in the country is Jose Visceral, known to most as Vice Ganda (Pamittan et al. 2017:95ff). Vice describes himself using the Tagalog term *bakla*, which means that he is a gay man, who also cross-dresses and shows gender expressions of a feminine or androgynous kind (ABS CBN News 2018). Another Tagalog word, *ganda*, which means 'beautiful', is likewise widely used by Filipinos who were assigned male at birth and identify as gay men, non-binary men, drag queens, cross-dressers and trans women. Perhaps the two most prominent *bakla*-identified people in

Narratives on Trans Health, Barriers to Care and Trans Sisterhood in the Philippines   195

the Philippines in the past decade would be Vice Ganda and Jennifer Laude, a trans woman who was murdered by a US marine in 2014. These two *gandas* have different narratives and perhaps even different ways of self-identification. They represent two different faces of trans experience in the Philippines.

There is no gender recognition law in the Philippines. There is also no same-sex union or marriage. The national SOGIE (sexual orientation, gender identities and expressions) Equality Bill, which was passed in August of 2019, was highly controversial, sparking weeks of debates and online discussions across the Philippines. At the height of this public discussion, a transpinay named Gretchen was disallowed from using the women's toilet in a mall in Quezon City. Gretchen incidentally was live on Facebook recording this event. She was publicly humiliated and embarrassed by how she was treated (Merez 2019).

The intervention of transpinay Congresswoman Geraldine Roman, as well as the cis allies senator Rissa Hontiveros and the mayor of Quezon City, Joy Belmonte, shifted the national debate on the SOGIE Equality Bill, an anti-discrimination ordinance which had been debated in various forms for twenty years (Talabong 2019). Most churches in the Philippines argued that such a law which 'tolerates' the LGBTIQ lifestyle should not be enacted. Nonetheless, the law was successfully passed in August 2019.

During these public debates, transphobic attitudes towards trans people using bathrooms according to their gender identity were widespread. Shockingly, many members of the LGBTIQ community either remained silent or showed no support for the enactment of the SOGIE Equality Bill. Some even rejected the bill, stating that LGBTIQ people, in general, should strive to blend in with the cis- and heteronormative lifestyle and should be grateful for being included.

Diane and *Pilar*: Hormone Use for Gender Affirmation Among Transpinays

The narratives and themes presented here draw on my graduate research which was conducted in the 2000s. I interviewed, observed and surveyed transpinays, hoping to understand many aspects of our identities, expressions and experiences.

Some experiences described by transpinays in my research project show the barriers to accessing hormone therapy:

"I don't know about medical supervision and it is scary because they might subject you to various laboratory tests. Plus, nobody told us about the word 'transitioning', we just know about hormones and the optional surgeries. Bottom line, if we can get it over the counter why go to the doctor?" – Trisha.

"Doctors are expensive, even more expensive than that box of pills. Why waste your money further?" – Ali.

"I was discouraged by a male doctor saying it is wrong and immoral to change my body as it is the temple of the Holy Spirit, of God. It violates God's rules on our creation. Since then, I realized I shouldn't consult a doctor on my hormone use, they just might stop me." – Frida.

Hormone intake has been known and widely spread amongst beauty pageants since the 1990s and gender-affirming surgeries have become more popular since the beginning of the 2000s. Among transpinays, when one talks about hormones, most would think of orally taken estrogen and/or progesterone. Mostly they were not aware, at least until the early 2000s, of the existence of patches and lotion gels and even now, seldom use intramuscular (IM) or injectable hormones.

Hormone therapy is not usually viewed in the Philippines as a component of medical transition that should be medically supervised (Alegre 2013). Rather, transpinays learned through parlor shop-talk and backstage chats at beauty pageants that the most feminine and beautiful among them were taking hormones on their own.

I, as a transpinay, could also relate to them. My interviews with transpinays and *baklas* showed a strong consensus within these communities that: (a) medical fees are expensive and there are administrative fees even for public hospitals, which have queues that last for hours; (b) Christian or catholic trained and raised doctors often invoke their religious beliefs to harass and discourage patients; and (c) it is not widely known that hormone use could be part of a transition package that is medically supervised.

Transpinays' unsupervised use of hormone medication reflects the broader prevalence of self-medication culture in the Philippines. One interviewee, Trisha, reported: "We self-medicate all the time, we use over the counter remedies and just ask the pharmacies what are alternatives and better doses to which they respond."

Although in recent years the local pharmacies have become stricter with over-the-counter drugs, self-medicating in consultation with pharmacists remains prevalent among Filipinos. Many medicines are endorsed by local celebrities. It is only more recently that concerns about liver and kidney damage due to over-medication are being addressed. The country has a long history with quack doctors, local herbologists and belief in the supernatural including witchcraft and voodoo. This cultural context may have some influence on the attitudes of transpinays today. There is also no medical benefit for the general public in the country comparable to the NHS of the UK or systems in Canada, US, Australia and EU. Hence many choose to take cheaper brands of hormones without understanding their varying effects and side effects. They may ingest oral contraceptives, estrogens or anti-androgens without necessarily knowing the difference. Further, intake and dosage of hormones varies considerably. Hormones are sometimes popped in like sweets:

"The more the merrier, hahaha, we just thought the more you take the faster your transformation will be. We just experience more headaches and tiredness, yet we feel more transformed. Although years later I realized, it's not the case, I still had to undergo top surgery for breasts..." – Frida.

The expectation that each hormone tablet contributes to feminization leads many transpinays to take very high doses. The more expensive the drugs are the less they take. The cheaper it is, or if it is freely available, the consumption increases. Cis women in some communities in the Philippines are given free access to oral contraceptive hormones and will sometimes provide these directly to their transpinay friends. Reproductive health is not well-practiced and lacks safe implementation in the Philippines since the church criticizes the principles of contraception and family planning (Alegre 2013). Therefore, many cis women pretend that they will take these pills and secretly give them to their transpinay friends.

Quick Change: Fillers and Silicone Injections

In contrast to expensive medically supervised and performed gender-affirming surgeries, since the mid-2000s, transpinays have learned about cheaper medical-grade fillers and silicone injections (Alegre 2013). Once more, most of this knowledge has been gained and spread throughout the pageant and parlor circles. Individuals who wish to undergo these procedures may look for someone amongst their peers who has experience injecting fillers and silicone, or they may learn to inject these themselves. The following quotes reflect some of the barriers to medically supervised procedures and attitudes toward these unofficial alternatives:

> "Women have these fuller face or higher cheekbones, more pointed chins and wider, fluffier hips and butts, and fillers and silicone injections are the only solution here. I will not do those surgeries, they're so expensive and scary." – Manda.

> "We met this girl who said she was trained as a nurse but could not afford to finish school and so she dropped out and became an aesthetician's assistant. She then became our supplier for fillers and silicone and she would come over to inject our faces, breasts and hips and butts." – Tasha.

It is unknown where this trend of fillers and silicone injections has started. Similar trends can be found amongst some communities of *travesties* in South America and amongst trans communities in South Korea and Thailand. It may be that transpinays have gained some knowledge about this practice overseas and introduced it to the local Philippine context.

Over time, the local community has used the expressions *chuk* and *tusha* to refer to injectable enhancers. This practice has become so prevalent that several widely viewed television programs have featured stories about these practices 'gone wrong'. Transpinays featured in these stories had some common life experiences. Many of them were poor, most worked for beauty parlors, some were beauty pageant contestants. All of them had the wish of appearing prettier and more feminine. They accessed these medically unsupervised treatments through their communities and weeks or months they suffered from side effects. Their faces showed bruises and lumps. The enhanced areas sagged and swelling never subsided (GMA 2017). The TV programs researching the stories worked together with medical doctors to reveal that many of these transpinays had been injected with industrial-grade silicon, which belongs in the automotive industry and should never be used for any type of body modification. These stories went viral and, as a result, medically approved fillers are becoming more popular. At the same time, some transpinays still use industrial silicone if they cannot afford more expensive fillers. Many of these transpinays are aware of the negative side effects, and that these could even be fatal, but will take the risk if it is the only option available to them. One transpinay beauty queen was famously quoted as saying:

"Dead, so be it, as long as I'm beautiful." – Yan Yan, Beauty Queen.

These stories of an unnamed, deceased transpinay queen inspired the well-received local films 'Die Beautiful' and 'Quick Change'. Both films featured the trans actress Mimi Juareza, who was awarded a Best Actor award. These films reflect the realities of transpinays in the Philippines: that self-medicated transition is a fearless and peer-trusting practice and, indeed, some would rather die beautiful than die masculine.

Summary and Recommendations: To Live Beautifully

Having taken into account the themes that emerged in my interviews over the years and my close interaction with other transpinays while living within the subculture of the Philippine queer movement, it is clear that the absence of gender recognition laws, medical plans and anti-discrimination laws have an impact on this community. In spite of these challenges, transpinays have found ways to navigate this exclusive system to fulfil their ideals of transitioning their bodies and selves. The lack of options within the medical system and the lack of acknowledgement of the presence of trans people and their health needs, has pushed many to bypass this system and to find affordable medically unsupervised treatments.

Another barrier to accessing medical care is the insufficient knowledge of medical professionals about the healthcare needs of trans people. Many doctors are not aware that Standards of Care, published by the World Association of Transgender Health, exist or even if they know, they are not willing to apply these standards. This creates an environment in which trans people avoid medical care altogether and resort to cultural practices of self-medication. Lack of acknowledgement within the Filipino medical system leads many trans people travel to Thailand for gender-affirming surgeries, where it is not only cheaper, but they can often access treatment faster than they would in the Philippines.

Transpinay health is likewise undermined by the absence of accessible medical information, for example information on pharmaceutical packaging that might be relevant to people who use these drugs for medical gender transition. As many transpinays say: if it is not written, it is not a rule.

Just as the Philippines' pre-colonial history was transmitted via oral tradition, trans healthcare practices today spread through word of mouth, at the community level. The relative absence of anti-discrimination laws forces some trans people to continue medically unsupervised transition practices, in order to "pass" in public. Yet, even if trans people can physically change to their desired appearance, their legal identity documents remain unchanged. This discrepancy adds to the oppression and violence that trans people experience day-to-day.

The two presented public figures, Vice Ganda and Jennifer Laude, are two representatives of queer identities in a catholic society like the Philippines. However, they are quite opposite. Vice is respected and adored as an entertainer. Their fame and fortune allow them to sail above most prejudices and stereotypes. Jennifer, on the other hand, was a survivor day-to-day. She was poor and ordinary. She had to survive in her small niche through sex work, which exposed her to additional risks of violence. Jennifer was murdered in October 2014 by a US marine. She because the face of hate crime in a country that relies on its colonial past and preaches how to live through the doctrines of the catholic church. To be *maganda*, or beautiful, in our country can be deadly.

There is a need for change on many levels. Structurally, the government of the Philippines must reconsider their stance on the SOGIE bill and to ensure it is enacted to protect the oppressed and invisible. On another level, the church must help to preach acceptance, instead of punishment. Medical institutions should find ways to include trans people in consultations and offer accessible language for treatment and procedures. Media should stop presenting queer people as objects of laughter and ridicule. Instead, it should move towards expansive and inclusive portrayals that reflect our authentic realities. Philippine society must reflect on the urgency of our needs to allow us to live our lives fully. Trans people should be more than just headlines in the daily news, where our stories range from being a beautiful feminine person in beauty pageants, to being victims of murder because allegedly we did not disclose our transness. There is much that needs to be done. At the end of the day, if society calls us *ganda* then at least we should be treated like it.

References

ABS CBN News (2018): Gay or transgender? Vice Ganda Gets Candid on sexual identity. In: ABS CBN News, 10 April 2018 [online]. Available at: https://news.abs-cbn.com/entertainment/04/10/18/gay-or-transgender-vice-ganda-gets-candid-on-sexual-identity (Accessed 15 November 2021).

Agilada, R. (2018): Roderick Paulate: Bading Nga Ba? In: Tempo Desk [online]. Available at: https://www.tempo.com.ph/2018/10/16/roderick-paulate-bading-ba/ (Accessed 15 November 2021).

Alegre, B. (2013): Toward a Better Understanding of Hormone and Silicone Injection use of Transgender Women in the Philippines and Hong Kong. Unpublished PhD Thesis. Santo Tomas: University of Santo Tomas.

Alegre, B. (2016): Psychological Perspectives of the Transsexual woman: A Phenomenological Case Study of Male to Female Transsexuals. Unpublished Master Thesis. Santo Tomas: University of Santo Tomas.

Associate Press (2016): Manny Pacquiao Apologizes for 'Gays worse than Animals' comment. In: Associated Press, 16 February 2016 [online]. Available at: https://www.scmp.com/sport/boxing/article/1913501/manny-pacquiao-apologises-same-sex-worse-animals-comment (Accessed 15 November 2021).

Brewer, C. (1999): Baylan, Asog, Transvestism and Sodomy: Gender, Sexuality and the Sacred in Early Colonial Philippines. In: Intersections: Gender, History and Culture in the Asian Context, 2(May 1999) [online]. Available at: http://intersections.anu.edu.au/issue2/carolyn2.html (Accessed 15 November 2021).

Call Her Granda (2019): Call Her Granda Timeline [online]. Available at: https://www.callherganda.com/jennifer-laudes-story/murder-case-timeline/ (Accessed 15 November 2021).

Corpuz, D. (2008): Subverting Zsazsa Zaturnah: A Critical Analysis on the Gender Representations on Carlo Vergara's Ang Kagilagilalas na Pakikipagsapalaran ni Zsazsa Zaturnah. Philippines: University of the Philippines.

Facial Injections Gone Wrong (2017). Directed by Kapuso Mo, Jessica Soho [Film]. Available at: https://en-gb.facebook.com/kapusomojessicasoho/videos/facial-injection-gone-wrong/10155119053041026/ (Accessed 15 November 2021).

Garcia, J., N. (1996): Philippine Gay Culture: Binabae to Bakla, Silahis to MSM. Philippines: University of the Philippines Press.

Inquirer News (2019): Baklang Hamburger?: Ricky Reyes Gives his Opinion on LGBT Issues. In: Inquirer News, 10 September 2019 [online]. Available at: https://entertainment.inquirer.net/344799/baklang-hamburger-ricky-reyes-gives-his-opinion-about-lgbt-issues (Accessed 15 November 2021).

Inton, M. (2017): The Bakla and the Silver Screen: Queer Cinema in the Philippines. PhD Thesis. Hong Kong: Lingnan University.

Johnson, J.M. (1997): Beauty and Power: Identity, Cultural Transformation and Transgendering in Southern Philippines. London: Routledge.

Merez, A. (2019): Pang parlor lang: Trans woman Gretchen Diez Hits Stereotypes. In: ABS CBN News, 16 August 2019 [online]. Available at: https://news.abs-cbn.com/news/08/16/19/pang-parlor-lang-trans-woman-gretchen-diez-hits-stereotypes (Accessed 15 November 2021).

Mosbergen, D. (2015): The Dangers of Being LGBT in 'Tolerant' Philippines. In: Huffington Post, 10 December 2015 [online]. Available at: https://www.huffpost.com/entry/lgbt-philippines_n_5614f92fe4b021e856d2d870 (Accessed 15 November 2021).

Nanda, S. (1998): Neither Man nor Woman: The Hijras of India. Belmont California: Wadsworth Publishing.

Pamittan, G.; Amaado, C.; Amante, V. and Demetrio, F. (2017): Kaloka, Keri, Bongga: Pakahulugan at Pahiwatig sa mga Piling Pelikula ni Vica Ganda. In: Plaridel Journal, 14(1, 2017), pp. 95-124.

PEW Research Centre (2013): The Global Divide on Homosexuality. Washinton, DC: PEW Research Centre. Available at: https://www.pewresearch.org/global/2013/06/04/the-global-divide-on-homosexuality/ (Accessed 15 November 2021).

Roscoe, W. (2016): Sexual and Gender Diversity in Native America and Pacific Islands. In: Springate, M. (Ed.): LGBTQ America: A Theme Study of Lesbian, Gay, Bisexual, Transgender and Queer History. Washington, DC: National Park Foundation, pp. 2- 27.

Sasot, S. (2012): Our Brave New World. In: Outrage Magazine, 17 November 2012 [online]. Available at: https://outragemag.com/our-brave-new-world-third-of-five/ (Accessed 15 November 2021).

Talabong, R. (2019): Energized by Gretchen Diez, Hontiveros renews push for SOGIE equality bill. In: Rappler, 14 August 2019 [online]. Available at: https://www.rappler.com/nation/hontiveros-renews-push-sogie-equality-bill-energized-gretchen-diez (Accessed 15 November 2021).

Tolentino, J. (2013): Those Crazy Coco B. Nights. In: Philippines Daily Inquirer, 29 September 2013 [online]. Available at: https://lifestyle.inquirer.net/127 965/those-crazy-coco-b-nights/ (Accessed 15 November 2021).

United Nations Development Programme and United States Agency for International Development (UNDP, USAID, 2014): Being LGBT in Asia: The Philippines Country Report [online]. Available at: https://pdf.usaid.gov/p df_docs/PBAAA888.pdf (Accessed 31 January 2022).

Dis-ease of Access: Health and Cancer Care Survey for Trans and Gender Diverse Australians

Lucille Kerr, Christopher M. Fisher & Tiffany Jones

Introduction

Drawing on results from a national survey involving 537 Trans and Gender Diverse (TGD) people, this chapter will focus on the experiences of TGD Australians accessing health and cancer care. The results document some of the diverse demographics of the TGD community in Australia, explore access to health and cancer care within the Australian context, and examine levels of awareness around cancer. The diversity includes many genders, sexualities, and backgrounds, whilst showing that TGD Australians remain a marginalized group that experiences much adversity. The data show that many TGD people have problems accessing healthcare due to experiences of mistreatment and ignorance on the part of providers – currently, access is plagued by dis-ease. Further, it appears that general awareness campaigns for cancer are not reaching this population. The recommendations offer ways forward through partnerships with TGD people themselves.

Social recognition and acceptance of TGD people is increasing in Australia. There has been an accompanying rapid rise in referrals for gender affirming care – some specialist clinics have seen their attendance multiply by ten in five years (2011-2016) (Cheung et al. 2018). Almost all of the specialized gender affirming care is provided by private professionals and there is a lack of funding and services (particularly outside of the major cities) (GLBTI Health and Wellbeing Ministerial Advisory Committee 2014; Telfer, Tollit and Feldman 2015). Research has documented that TGD people in Australia experience high rates of marginalization and discrimination in the general community, with poor mental health and an increase in detrimental health behaviors (e.g., smoking) as a likely consequence (Hyde et al. 2014; Smith et al. 2014). Limited pathways to surgery mean that TGD people often have body parts and organs which cause them significant distress (GLBTI Health and Wellbeing Ministerial Advisory Committee 2014). Such distress can act as an additional barrier to accessing healthcare and cancer screening services. However, the more significant barriers appear to be the mistreatment commonly experienced by this community and the lack of awareness within the healthcare system (Jones et al. 2015; Riggs and Due 2013). Many TGD people have a strong and justified fear of mistreatment and may avoid services as a result. The paucity of research addressing this issue is a further exacerbation, as even gender affirmation specialists may find themselves unable to make evidence-based decisions or enact change due to the lack of data. Additionally, population-based research and registries do not include information on diverse genders. Subsequently, there is a lack of consideration in policies and allocation of resources (Ansara 2016). This chapter will outline a national Australian study of TGD people that explored their experiences of accessing health and cancer care, providing background, methodology, results, discussion, conclusion and recommendations.

Social, Health and Care Experiences of TGD Australians

Australian research has established that TGD people experience a variety of adverse circumstances due to social marginalization and stigmatization. For example, TGD Australians are generally well-educated, yet this is not reflected in their income or employment rates, with significantly lower income and levels of employment than both the general and (cis) gay, lesbian, and bisexual population (Boza and Nicholson-Perry 2014; Jones et al. 2015; Hyde et al. 2014). They are also at a greater risk of homelessness, frequently encounter familial rejection, and are likely to be socially isolated, especially if they live outside of a metropolitan area (Jones et al. 2015; McNair et al. 2017; Riggs, Ansara and Treharne 2015). Up to 87.4% of TGD Australians report having experienced discrimination based on their gender (Couch et al. 2007). Areas of discrimination include social/community, employment, economic and family, and may be in the form of verbal, written, physical, sexual, or exclusory actions (Beyond Blue 2012). A range of lifestyle behaviors that may influence cancer risk have also been found in relatively high rates including: smoking, alcohol abuse, and limiting exercise due to discomfort (intense exercising may be dangerous for people who use chest binders) (Boza and Nicholson-Perry 2014; Hyde et al. 2014; Smith et al. 2014). Higher rates of poor mental health when compared with the general population have been documented, with depression found to be up to four times that of the general population (Hyde et al. 2014). Arguably, the three main factors that determine mental health for TGD Australians are discrimination, access to gender affirming technologies, and social/familial support (Riggs, Ansara and Treharne 2015).

Documentation is another issue that may have wide-ranging effects on TGD Australians' lives. The process of changing one's identifying documents may be a vital step in recognition of their gender (Hyde et al. 2014; Jones et al. 2015). In Australia, different identity documents may be under Commonwealth or state/territory legislation, meaning there are varying requirements, some of which have an unreasonably high burden of proof (e.g., the requirement to have had gender affirming surgery to change one's birth certificate) (GLBTI Health and Wellbeing Ministerial Advisory Committee 2014). Many in the TGD community report being unable to change some or all of their documentation as a result (Hyde et al. 2014). Inability to change documentation may expose them to discrimination and lead to poorer health and wellbeing.

Another factor to consider in relation to the diversity and health of TGD Australians is intersectionality, particularly as it relates to the experiences of Aboriginal and Torres Strait Islander People. Indigenous communities in Australia have experienced ongoing trauma and adversity since colonization began in 1788, including loss of life to infectious disease, violence, forced relocation, and breakdowns in family and community due to the government-sanctioned removal of children from their parents (Kerry 2014). Aboriginal and Torres Strait Islander people suffer considerable disadvantage and, as a result, poorer physical and mental health, with a life expectancy ten years less than the general Australian population (Australian Institute of Health and Welfare 2018). Sistergirl and brotherboy are indigenous Australian terms for two distinct gender identifications – although the terms are not equivalent, sistergirl aligns with trans woman, and brotherboy with trans man (Kerry 2014). Sistergirls, brotherboys and other Aboriginal and Torres Strait Islander people who experience some form of gender diversity, may face significant challenges to their health and wellbeing, and marginalization due to cultural difference may further complicate their access to healthcare. Whilst efforts were made throughout this study to encourage participation of Aboriginal and Torres Strait Islander people, unfortunately there was not a sufficient proportion of the sample to run statistical tests for comparison. This reflects the difficulties in recruiting a culturally diverse sample on a limited time-line and budget, as well as the broader context of ongoing marginalization of Aboriginal and Torres Strait Islander people in Australian society.

For those who can safely access it, Australia is fortunate to have a health-care system that is one of the most affordable and comprehensive in the world (Lowe and Cristofis 2017). A complicated combination of both public and private, the system includes national subsidy schemes for medical pro-cedures (Medicare Benefits Schedule), medications (Pharmaceutical Benefits Scheme), and private health insurance (Australian Government Rebate on Pri-vate Health Insurance) (Lowe and Cristofis 2017). For TGD people, access to subsidies may be limited due to these being 'gendered', and the fact that some gender affirming surgeries are either partly or wholly labelled as 'cosmetic' (GLBTI Health and Wellbeing Ministerial Advisory Committee 2014). Addi-tionally, gatekeeping by healthcare professionals, particularly psychiatrists, is a stressful process for many TGD people and is another barrier to accessing gender affirming care (Ho and Mussap 2017). Gatekeeping may relate to hor-mones and/or surgery and involves the healthcare professional assessing the individual to see if they meet the criteria for the interventions sought with the goal being to obtain a 'letter' of approval so they may proceed with gender affirming care (ibid.). Australia is a sparsely populated country, with most of its population living in two highly urbanized coastal areas that are widely sep-arated (Australian Bureau of Statistics 2012). Access to healthcare services is especially a problem for those who live rurally/remotely, with increased travel, accommodation and financial burdens (GLBTI Health and Wellbeing Minis-terial Advisory Committee 2014).

Australian research has found a lack of TGD sensitive services, inadequate knowledge on the part of healthcare professionals, problems with access, and a high frequency of bad experiences which result in avoidance of healthcare and poor mental health (Couch et al. 2007; Hyde et al. 2014; McLean 2011; Riggs and Due 2013; Strauss et al. 2017). The characteristics of bad experi-ences for TGD Australians include; lack of respect; expressions of hostility, surprise, discomfort, contempt, and disgust; prejudicial attitudes; misgen-dering language; the patient having to educate the healthcare professional; refusal of services; and feeling pathologized (Ho and Mussap 2016; Jones et al. 2015; McLean 2011; Riggs and Due 2013). Couch et al. (2007) found that many TGD people are not fully expressing themselves in healthcare, and Smith et al. (2014) reported that only 6% of their participants who experienced mis-treatment had made a complaint about it. Due to the negative experiences of themselves and others in their community, many TDG people are understandably reluctant to access services or disclose their gender, which results in unmet needs and the potential to miss serious illnesses or care requirements. Cancer care itself may be especially difficult due since public health messaging about common types of cancer, for example breast and prostate, is usually highly gendered (Kerr and Jones 2017).

In their important role for primary healthcare, General Practitioners (GPs) are often the first point of contact when engaging with health services. GPs provide ongoing support and care, make referrals to more specialized care (and may be seen as 'gatekeepers' for this reason), and coordinate the care of their patients (Strauss et al. 2017). GPs are the most common healthcare professional for people to access in relation to their gender, and an individual's health needs are more likely to be met if they have a good, regular general practitioner (Hyde et al. 2014; Strauss et al. 2017). In 2014, Hyde et. al. found that only half of their TGD participants that had a regular GP met the criteria for a 'good' doctor-patient relationship. TGD people may have varied experiences with GPs due to the heterogeneity of different clinicians' knowledge and attitudes.

In terms of access to healthcare, it has been found that TGD Australians do not feel that they are having their health needs met (Hyde et al. 2014). Both the government and private sectors are seen to be inadequate to meet the needs of this population, under-funded, and not coping with the demand for gender affirmative care which results in long waiting periods for many individuals (ibid.). Ideally, an individual should be able to choose who provides their healthcare, but currently there are insufficient services for this to be the case for most TGD Australians.

The overarching aims of this study were to explore the experiences of TGD people in health and cancer care, including factors that prevent or promote access. Specific research questions include 'is having unmet healthcare needs associated with more barriers to care?' and which factors may predict barriers to care. The next section details methodology, including survey design, recruitment, and administration.

Study Methodology and Design

This study used a community-based participatory research design to conduct an online survey (Adams et al. 2017; Hacker 2017). The community was consulted and involved throughout, including during the survey design, recruitment, analysis and reporting. Additionally, key informant interviews were conducted with TGD community members and professionals that had relevant knowledge to guide development of the research (for further detail see Kerr, Fisher and Jones 2019).

Participants and Procedure:

A convenience sample was recruited through paid online Facebook advertising and TGD community promotion (generating a snowball sample). A total of 854 surveys were saved, one third of which were incomplete surveys. Data cleaning removed 21 responses which were illegitimate (e.g., mischievous responders), leaving 537 participants. Average completion time for the survey was 22 minutes. The mean age of participants was 26.64 (SD = 10.93, range 18-79). Participants' genders were 22.7% (n=122) trans women, 33.0% (n=177) trans men and 44.3% (n=238) gender diverse people. For sex assigned at birth, 70.9% (n=381) were assigned female at birth and 26.6% (n=143) assigned male at birth, with 2.4% (n=13) choosing not to disclose. Of the sample, 6.3% (n=26) reported that they were Aboriginal or Torres Strait Islander. More participant socio-demographics are detailed in the results section.

Measures:

The survey covered four areas: socio-demographics, gender affirmation, accessing healthcare, and cancer awareness and care. Questions were forced-choice, containing 'prefer not to answer' options, and there were text boxes at many points to provide qualitative comments. The number of questions asked of each participant varied as some sections were open only to people who had specific body organs (e.g., a cervix). To allow for comparisons with the general Australian population and international TGD communities, measures were taken from the 2016 Australian Census, the Australian Bureau of Statistics Survey of Healthcare, the Cancer Awareness Measure and other TGD research (e.g., experiences of discrimination from the Canadian Trans PULSE study and bad experiences in healthcare from the 2015 U.S. Transgender Survey).

The Kessler 6 (K6) uses six items to assess levels of general psychological distress (Kessler et al. 2002). Feelings of nervousness, hopelessness, restlessness, depression, effort and worthlessness in the past 30 days are rated on a five-point Likert scale from 'none of the time' to 'all of the time' (ibid.). Scores range from 0-24, with a score over 13 being indicative of probable mental illness (ibid.). The K6 is a reliable tool for measuring psychological distress.

Barriers to care were measured using seven out of ten items from the 'Barriers to Help Seeking' section of the Cancer Awareness Measure (Stubbings et al. 2009). Added to these seven items were two items developed by the team that are specific to TGD Australians ('fear of mistreatment' and 'unable to find a doctor I am comfortable with'). The question was 'do any of the following things stop you from going to the doctor?', with potential answers being 'no', 'sometimes' and 'often'. A Barriers to Care Score was created summing the nine items, with scores ranging from 0-18. The Barriers to Care Score is a key measure for analyses in this chapter.

Analysis:

SPSS V25 was used to analyze the data. Descriptive statistics were run for selected key socio-demographics, gender affirmation, access to healthcare, and cancer care and awareness. Researchers then wanted to answer the question 'is having unmet healthcare needs associated with more barriers to care?' A t-test was run to compare the Barriers to Care Score between the two groups of those who reported having an unmet healthcare need and those who did not. Additionally, researchers wanted to know what factors influenced Barriers to Care Scores. For this reason, a standard multiple regression was conducted to see if the five measures of age, sex assigned at birth, income, K6 score, and number of bad experiences in healthcare predicted Barriers to Care Scores, how much variance could be explained by these factors, and which of these factors is the best at predicting barriers to care.

Results: Sociodemographic, Barriers to Care and Healthcare Experiences

Tables 1-5 display descriptive results for socio-demographic characteristics, health, psychological distress, gender affirmation, barriers to care, experiences of participants accessing healthcare, and cancer care and awareness. The majority of participants were trans men or non-binary, under the age of 25, single, had very low income, and identified as pansexual and/or bisexual. Most participants rated their health as either fair or good, reported high levels of psychological distress, experienced multiple forms of discrimination, had not been able to change all of their identifying documents, and attended a doctor for gender affirmation in the last 12 months. The mean for the K6 score was 12.53. The most common barriers to care were too many other things to worry about, inability to find a doctor they are comfortable with, being too busy, and fear of mistreatment. The mean for the Barriers to Care Score was 6.62. In terms of healthcare experiences, most participants reported that they had an unmet healthcare need (mostly due to cost and fear of mistreatment), were very uncomfortable discussing their needs with a healthcare provider that they do not know, only disclosed their gender to a healthcare provider if they had to and have had to teach a Healthcare Worker (HCW) about TGD people to get appropriate care. Cancer awareness was generally low to moderate, with the majority of participants reporting that a HCW had not discussed cancer topics with them.

Tests of the Research Questions

An independent-samples t-test was conducted to compare the Barriers to Care Score for those who reported ever having an unmet healthcare need (58.8%, n=300) and those who did not (41.2%, n=210). Participants who ever had an unmet healthcare need reported significantly more barriers to care (Mean = 7.69) than those who indicated they did not have an unmet healthcare need (Mean = 4.98).

Standard multiple regression was used to assess whether age, sex assigned at birth, income (dichotomous, ≤$37,000 and $37,001+), K6 score, and bad experiences in healthcare predict the Barriers to Care Score. The variance explained by this model was 32.7%, meaning that almost a third of Barriers to Care are explained by these five factors. Four variables were statistically significant, with the K6 score being of highest significance, followed by bad experiences in healthcare, age, and sex assigned at birth. Income was not statistically significant. Higher Barriers to Care Scores were predicted by higher psychological distress, more bad experiences in healthcare, being younger, and assigned female at birth.

Table 1: Sociodemographic Characteristics of the Sample.

Gender		
Woman	31	5.8%
Man	26	4.8%
Trans woman	90	16.8%
Trans man	146	27.2%
Genderqueer	32	6.0%
Non-binary	142	26.4%
Gender-fluid	29	5.4%
Agender	11	2.0%
Something else	30	5.6%
Age		
18-24	326	60.7%
25-34	110	20.5%
35-44	59	11.0%
45+	42	7.8%
Relationship Status		
Single and not dating	210	39.7%
Single and dating	61	11.5%
Partnered, not living together	209	20.6%
Partnered, living together	131	24.8%
Polyamorous/open relationship	18	3.4%
Individual Income before Tax (AUD)		
$0-$18,200	282	57.6%
$18,201-$37,000	89	18.2%
$37,001-$87,000	91	18.6%
$87,001-$180,000	28	5.7%
Sexuality (multiple response answer)		
Heterosexual	40	9.4%
Gay	61	14.4%
Bisexual	129	30.4%
Lesbian	61	14.4%

Pansexual	150		35.4%
Queer	44		10.4%
Asexual	89		21.0%
Experienced Homelessness		130	31.3%
Disclosed an Area of Neurodiversity		152	38.0%
Disclosed a Disability		103	25.8%
Engagement with the TGD Community			
Never, rarely or yearly		144	34.4%
Monthly		56	13.4%
Daily or weekly		219	52.3%

Table 2: Health, Psychological Distress and Gender Affirmation

Self-reported Health		
Poor	68	12.7%
Fair	176	32.8%
Good	178	33.2%
Very good	96	17.9%
Excellent	18	3.4%
K6 Dichotomous		
High levels of psychological distress	280	52.2%
Low levels of psychological distress	256	47.8%
Experiences of Discrimination		
Silent harassment	455	84.7%
Verbal harassment	382	71.1%
Physical intimidation and threats	199	37.1%
Physical violence	105	19.6%
Sexual harassment	232	43.2%
Sexual Assault	155	28.9%
None of the above	47	8.8%
Changing Identity Documents		

Do not want to	72	13.7%
Have not but plan to in future	196	37.4%
Unable to	82	15.6%
Able to change some	120	22.9%
Changed all documentation	54	10.3%
Hormone Use		
Never taken hormones	247	46.7%
Previously on hormones	18	3.4%
Currently on hormones	244	46.1%
On hormones for medical reasons	20	3.8%
Had Surgery	115	21.9%
Seen a Doctor for Gender Affirmation in the Last 12 Months	303	56.6%
Inability to Access Gender Affirming Care (last 12 months)*	181	43.2%

*Excludes those not desiring access to gender affirming care.

Table 3: Barriers to Care.

	No		Sometimes		Of-ten
	n	%	n	%	n
Fear of mistreatment	219	41.2%	235	44.3%	77
Unable to find doctor I'm comfortable with	165	31.1%	220	41.5%	145
I find my doctor difficult to talk to	245	46.0%	204	38.3%	84
Difficult to make an appointment	239	45.2%	176	33.3%	114
I am too busy	215	40.4%	203	38.2%	114
I do not have money to see the doctor	263	49.3%	166	31.1%	104
Too many other things to worry about	156	29.3%	240	45.1%	136
Difficult to arrange transport to the doctor	329	61.6%	135	25.3%	70
Worrying about what the doctor might find	296	55.3%	161	30.1%	78

Table 4: Healthcare Experiences.

Unmet Healthcare Need (ever)	300	58.8%
Unmet Healthcare Need (last 12 months)	242	47.5%
Reasons for Unmet Healthcare Needs*		
Financial cost	138	46.0%
Fear of disrespect/mistreatment	133	44.3%
Could not get an appointment	105	35.0%
No nearby services	46	15.3%
Refused services due to being TGD	24	8.0%
Comfort Discussing Needs with a Healthcare Provider They Do Not Know		
Very uncomfortable	237	44.5%
Uncomfortable	196	36.8%
Comfortable	87	16.4%
Very Comfortable	12	2.3%
Information Needs Related to Care**		
Have not received enough information	137	36.8%
Have received enough information	235	63.2%
Did Not Have a Healthcare Provider with a Good Understanding of Their Needs, Preferences (last 12 months)***	129	26.9%
Multiple Attempts to Access Appropriate Healthcare (last 12 months)		
Sometimes	225	44.6%
Often	73	14.5%
Worsening Health due to the Length of Time Taken to get Appropriate Care		
Sometimes	166	32.7%
Often	62	12.2%
Needed Emergency Care but Avoided Attending the Emergency Department because they were Trans or Gender Diverse	144	41.3%
Disclosing Gender to Healthcare Workers		
Never	65	12.2%
Only if I have to	225	42.4%
Sometimes	110	20.7%
Always	66	12.4%

I do not have a choice (documentation shows this)	65	12.2%
Never had a HCW know they were TGD and treat them with respect	133	26.5%
Had to teach HCW about TGD people so they could get appropriate care	279	55.6%
HCW refused to give them gender affirming care	115	23.0%
HCW refused to give them general healthcare	106	20.7%
HCW asked them unnecessary/invasive questions related to being TGD not related to the reason for their visit	194	37.7%
HCW has used harsh or abusive language when treating them	80	15.4%
HCW was physically rough or abusive when treating them	30	5.7%
Experienced verbal harassment in a healthcare setting	74	14.2%
Have been physically attacked in a healthcare setting	12	2.3%
Experienced unwanted sexual contact in a healthcare setting	30	5.7%

*Percentages based on those who reported having an unmet healthcare need.
**Excludes those who had no information needs.
***Excludes those who had no healthcare needs.

Table 5: Cancer Care and Awareness

How soon would you see a HCW if you had a cancer symptom		
I would not make an appointment	41	9.8%
Within a year	31	7.4%
Within a few months	86	20.6%
Within a month	76	18.2%
Within a week	46	11.0%
As soon as possible	138	33.0%
HCW has not discussed cancer topics with them	260	60.5%
HCW recommendation of cervical screening*		

Never	155	56.8%
Once	69	25.3%
Often	49	17.9%
Accessed cervical screening*		
Never	163	58.7%
Once or rarely		
Regularly	43	15.8%

Cancer Awareness Items (frequencies for correct responses)		
Hormones can affect everyone's cancer risk (*true*).	191	44.6%
The risk of getting cancer does not increase with age (*false*).	324	75.5%
It is not necessary to have screening for cervical cancer if someone with a cervix has never been sexually active in any way (*true*).	42	9.8%
The Australian cervical cancer screening program has recently changed (*true*).	143	33.4%
People who are assigned male at birth cannot develop breast cancer (*false*).	392	91.8%
People do not have any risk of developing breast cancer if they have had a mastectomy (*false*).	263	61.7%
People with breasts/chest tissue between the ages of 50 and 74 should have a mammogram once every two years (*true*).	314	73.4%
Australia has a nation-wide breast cancer screening program (*true*).	286	66.8%
Australia has a nation-wide prostate cancer screening program (*false*).	19	4.4%
Australia has a nation-wide bowel screening program (*true*).	220	51.4%

*Note: Excludes people who do not have a cervix.

Discussion

This chapter has presented a snapshot of TGD Australians accessing health and cancer care, including analyses around barriers to care. The data builds on findings from previous Australian research, whilst shedding further light on the issues facing TGD people accessing care. As the study shows, Australia has a diverse TGD community, who have various genders (many of which are outside of the binary), many sexual identities, and different backgrounds. The sample was overall young, and many are engaging frequently with others in the TGD population, indicating a strong and evolving community who potentially feel safer to be visible. These are aspects of our participants' experiences that are heartening and offer much hope for empowerment into the future. On the other hand, social stigma and marginalization clearly remain a significant and pressing issue. Of note, and consistent with previous research, our participants had low incomes, high rates of having experienced homelessness, and multiple experiences of discrimination and assault (Hyde et al. 2014). The follow-on from this is high levels of psychological distress and poorer health when compared with the general Australian population. Over half (52.2%) of the sample fell into the range of 'probable serious mental illness' using the Kessler 6, whereas Australian data using the Kessler 10 shows that 11.7% of the general Australian population fall into this category (Australian Bureau of Statistics 2015). Very few people (3.4%) in our sample reported 'excellent' health – this is much lower than the general Australian population, of which 20% have been found to rate they health as excellent (ibid.).

Neurodiversity was reported by well over a third of the sample, with other research supporting a relatively high rate of neurodiversity for TGD people (Strauss et al. 2017). This is significant for healthcare providers to note, as navigating healthcare may be difficult for people who are neurodiverse, with many healthcare professionals lacking knowledge and awareness of appropriate care (Lehmann and Leavey 2017). Further to this, experiences of physical and sexual assault are not uncommon, meaning that TGD people are more likely to have trauma histories. In addition to care that is inclusive for people who are neurodiverse, trauma-informed care is an important step in making services sensitive to TGD people's needs. This involves sensitive screening for a trauma history, developing trusting relationships, minimizing distress, and maximizing autonomy (Reeves 2015). Extending this person-centered care also means addressing an individual's body discomfort, and healthcare providers having an awareness of how and when to ask the right questions about sex organs (*without* being unnecessarily invasive), which is especially important given that most TGD people do not always disclose their gender to healthcare workers.

Given that in Australia the legislation related to various identifying documents may be under state/territory or federal government administration, and the requirements therefore are not consistent, it is unsurprising that the data shows difficulty changing documentation. There is diversity in how TGD people choose to medically affirm their gender, with many choosing to use hormones, however, rates of surgery appear to be relatively low. Partly this is likely because of the young age of our cohort as people are more likely to have surgery the older, they are due to financial circumstances, but in addition to this surgery in Australia is limited and difficult to access (GLBTI Health and Wellbeing Ministerial Advisory Committee 2014). Many (43.2%) of our participants reported that there was a time in the last year they wanted to access gender affirmation but were unable to. This provides further evidence that there are not enough services to meet current demands.

Almost half of our participants said that there was a time they needed healthcare in the past year but did not receive it, which is twice that seen in the general Australian population (Australian Bureau of Statistics 2017). That many say that this is because of cost shows there is still a financial burden associated with accessing healthcare, despite coverage for many aspects of this in Australia. This financial cost could relate to getting time off work and travel and may also be associated with the fact that many gender affirmation specialists are within the private health system. Significantly, 44.3% said they had an unmet healthcare need because they were afraid, they would be disrespected or mistreated, which fits with the high rate of bad experiences in healthcare. Unsurprisingly, few people are comfortable discussing their needs with healthcare workers that they do not know. Over a quarter of participants reported not receiving enough information about their care in the last year, which is more than three times that found in the general Australian population (ibid.). Additionally, just under a quarter said that they did not have a healthcare provider with a good understanding of their needs – considerably higher than the 9% found in the general Australian population (ibid.). The survey results consistently demonstrate that healthcare services and workers are not equitable for TGD people.

There were a range of bad experiences reported by our participants. Over a quarter had never had a healthcare provider know they were TGD and treat them with respect. Over half have had to educate their healthcare provider, almost a quarter have been refused gender affirming care, one fifth have been refused general healthcare, and over a third have had a healthcare provider ask unnecessary questions about their gender unrelated to their visit. In this context, there is complete legitimacy to TGD people's fears of mistreatment. This also reflects the lack of knowledge on the part of healthcare workers and indicates a need for further training.

The analyses around barriers to care show that there are numerous things preventing TGD people from accessing care. For seven out of nine of these barriers, over half of participants reported that these items either 'sometimes' or 'often' stopped them from going to the doctor. The items with the most people indicating they 'sometimes' or 'often' stopped them from going to the doctor were as follows: 'too many other things to worry about' (70.7%); 'unable to find a doctor I am comfortable with' (68.9%); 'I am too busy' (59.6%); 'fear of mistreatment' (58.8%); 'difficult to make an appointment' (54.8%); 'I find my doctor difficult to talk to' (54.0%); and 'I do not have money to see the doctor' (50.7%). TGD people have multiple stressors in their lives, including low income and experiences of discrimination, and it is therefore unlikely that making an appointment to see the doctor takes priority. Additionally, their bad experiences as detailed above are affecting their access because they are fearful of what they will encounter in a healthcare setting. Having more barriers to care is associated with unmet healthcare needs, as shown in the T-test.

Approximately one out of six participants reported that they either would not make an appointment or would delay this up to a year if they had a symptom that they thought was a sign of cancer. That the problems accessing healthcare result in a such a serious outcome shows how fearful TGD people are of healthcare environments. Delaying seeking medical attention this long for a cancer symptom is likely to result in higher morbidity and mortality for this community. Other issues in relation to cancer care are that healthcare providers are not discussing the topic with TGD people, and as shown by the generally low awareness levels (table 4), general cancer awareness campaigns do not reach TGD people. There is a need for more focused attention in this area; the TGD population should be a priority group for cancer organizations and specific awareness campaigns should be designed for them. Likewise, mainstream cancer awareness campaigns should stop relying on gendered messaging that actively excludes TGD people.

For participants who have a cervix, the results show that healthcare providers are not recommending cervical screening to them – over half said this had never happened, and a further quarter said this had happened only once. Partly this can be attributed to the young age of the sample (in Australia guidelines state for cervical screening to begin at age 21). However, it is also likely that healthcare providers are making assumptions based on TGD people's appearances, that they are not asking the right questions, and that TGD people are hesitant to disclose information about their bodies. A small percentage of TGD people with a cervix reported being regular screeners, but over half reported that they had never had cervical screening. Cervical cancer is an extremely preventable disease with screening, and moreover, the biggest risk factor for developing it is not attending screening (Johnson et al. 2016). Healthcare providers and cancer screening awareness campaigns need to be actively including TGD people with a cervix, ensuring that they know that this screening is relevant and important for them.

The findings from the standard multiple regression indicate that, taken together, higher levels of psychological distress, bad experiences in healthcare, younger age and being assigned female at birth significantly predict barriers to care. Research that has examined TGD people delaying care because of fear of mistreatment has found that this results in poorer mental health (Seelman et al. 2017). It is unsurprising that having bad experiences within healthcare is a significant predictor for increased barriers to care, as TGD Australians' expectations are likely to be based on their own and others' everyday lived experience. The results may indicate a trend that as TGD people grow older, they have had more time to find a sensitive healthcare provider, thus they have fewer barriers. People who were assigned female at birth may find the prospect of accessing care difficult since those certain procedures (e.g., cervical screening) may be especially invasive and uncomfortable for them. Income was not a significant predictor for barriers to care, which may reflect the fact that Australia's health system is largely affordable. Overall, the data demonstrate clearly that accessing health and cancer care as a TGD person can be very difficult.

Conclusion & Recommendations

The TGD community in Australia is diverse, evolving and strong. However, there is ongoing social marginalization, stigma and experiences of violence, and much work to be done to improve the situation. This survey found numerous, wide-ranging examples of problems related to accessing health and cancer care. There is a critical need for widespread training and education of people working within the healthcare system, and patient-centered care that is appropriate for people with neurodiversity and trauma histories. Enhanced coverage and accessibility are needed for gender affirmation services, which are currently insufficient to meet demand. The recommendations are as follows:

1. The data strongly support a person-centered approach to health and cancer care for TGD individuals, which considers gender, bodies, neurodi-

versity and trauma histories. Healthcare workers need to be initiating the relevant conversations in a sensitive manner and tailoring their care appropriately.

2. There is a need for widespread training and education, including in prevocational courses for medicine, nursing, and allied health.
3. Health and cancer policies should make TGD people a priority population.
4. Changes need to be made regarding the ways in which population-based research and registries collect gender/sex information.
5. Gender affirmation services need increased funding to ensure accessibility.
6. There is a need for general cancer awareness campaigns to be more inclusive of TGD people and also a need for specific TGD campaigns.
7. Health and cancer care need to make partnerships with the TGD community to develop guidelines and interventions to improve care.

Health and cancer care must make the TGD population a priority group, and population-based data collection needs to change in order to get a better picture on what is happening for this community. The dis-ease of access is in need of comprehensive treatment.

References

Adams, N.; Pearce, R.; Veale, J.; Radix, A.; Castro, D.; Sarkar, A.; and Thom, K.C. (2017): Guidance and Ethical Considerations for Undertaking Transgender Health Research and Institutional Review Boards Adjudicating this Research. In: Transgender Health, 2(1), pp. 165-175.

Ansara, G. (2016): Making the Count: Addressing data integrity gaps in Australian standards for collecting sex & gender. Newtown: National LGBTI Health Alliance.

Australian Bureau of Statistics (ABS, 2012): Year Book Australia, 2012. Canberra: Commonwealth Government of Australia.

Australian Bureau of Statistics (ABS, 2015): National Health Survey: First results. Australia 2014-15. Canberra: Commonwealth Government of Australia.

Australian Bureau of Statistics (ABS, 2017): Survey of Healthcare, Australia 2016. Canberra: Commonwealth Government of Australia.

Australian Institute of Health and Welfare (AIHW, 2018): Deaths in Australia. Web report [online]. Available at: https://www.aihw.gov.au/reports/life-e xpectancy-death/deaths/ (Accessed: 11 November 2021).

Bariola, E.; Lyons, A.; Leonard, W.; Pitts, M.; Badcock, P. and Couch, M. (2015): Demographic and Psychosocial Factors Associated With Psychological Distress and Resilience Among Transgender Individuals. In: Journal of Public Health, 105(10), pp. 2108-2116.

Bauer, G. and Scheim, A. (2015): Transgender People in Ontario, Canada: Statistics to Inform Human Rights Policy. Ontario: University of Western Ontario.

Beyond Blue (2012): In My Shoes: Experiences of discrimination, depression & anxiety among gay, lesbian, bisexual, trans and intersex people. Hawthorn: Beyond Blue.

Boza, C. and Nicholson-Perry, K. (2014): Gender-Related Victimisation, Perceived Social Support, and Predictors of Depression Among Transgender Australians. In: International Journal of Transgenderism, 15(1), pp. 35-52.

Cheung, A.; Ooi, O.; Leemaqz, S.; Cundill, P.; Silberstein, N.; Bretherton, I.; Thrower, E.; Locke, P.; Grossmann, M. and Zajac, J. (2018): Sociodemographic and Clinical Characteristics of Transgender Adults in Australia. In: Transgender Health, 3(1), pp. 229-238.

Couch, M.; Pitts, M.; Mulcare, H.; Croy, S.; Mitchell, A. and Patel, S. (2007): TranZnation: A report on the health and wellbeing of transgender people in Australia and New Zealand. Melbourne: ARCSHS, La Trobe University.

GLBTI Health and Wellbeing Ministerial Advisory Committee (2014): Transgender and Gender Diverse Health and Wellbeing. Melbourne: Victorian Department of Health.

Hacker, K. (2017): Community-Based Participatory Research. London: Sage Publications Ltd.

Ho, F. and Mussap, A. (2017): Transgender Mental Health in Australia: Satisfaction with Practitioners and the Standards of Care. In: Australian Psychologist, 52(3), pp. 209-218.

Hyde, Z.; Doherty, M.; Tilley, M.; McCaul, K.; Kieran; Rooney, R. and Jancey, J. (2014): The First Australian National Trans Mental Health Study: Summary of Results. Perth: School of Public Health, Curtin University.

James, S.; Herman, J.; Rankin, S.; Keisling, M.; Mottet, L. and Anafi, M. (2016): Executive Summary of the Report of the 2015 U.S. Transgender Survey. Washington D.C.: National Center for Transgender Equality.

Johnson, M.; Mueller, M.; Eliason, M.; Stuart, G. and Nemeth, L. (2016): Qualitative and mixed analyses to identify factors that affect cervical cancer screening uptake among lesbian and bisexual women and transgender men. In: Journal of Clinical Nursing, 25(23-24), pp. 3628-3642.

Jones, T.; del Pozo de Bolger, A.; Dune, T.; Lykins, A. and Hawkes, G. (2015): Female-to-Male (FtM) Transgender People's Experiences in Australia: A National Study. Switzerland: Springer International Publishing.

Kerr, L. and Jones, T. (2017): Cancer Screening for Trans and Gender Diverse People. In: Jones, T. (Ed.): Bent Street. Melbourne: Clouds of Magellan Press, pp. 25-35.

Kerr, L.; Fisher, C.M. and Jones, T. (2019): TRANScending Discrimination in Health and Cancer Care: A Study of Trans and Gender Diverse Australians. ARCSHS Monograph Series No. 115. Melbourne: Australian Research Centre in Sex, Health and Society, La Trobe University.

Kerry, S. (2014): Sistergirls/Brotherboys: The Status of Indigenous Transgender Australians. In: International Journal of Transgenderism, 15, pp. 173-186.

Kessler, R.C.; Andrews, G.; Colpe, L.J.; Hiripi, E.; Mroczek, D.K.; Normand, S.L.T.; Walters, E.E. and Zaslavsky, A.M. (2002): Short screening scales to monitor population prevalences and trends in non-specific psychological distress. In: Psychological Medicine, 32(6), pp. 959-976.

Lehmann, K. and Leavey, G. (2017): Individuals with gender dysphoria and autism: barriers to good clinical practice. In: Journal of Psychiatric and Mental Health Nursing, 24(2-3), pp. 171-177.

Leonard, W.; Pitts, M.; Mitchell, A.; Lyons, A.; Smith, A.; Patel, S.; Couch, M. and Barrett, A. (2012): Private Lives 2: The second national survey of the health and wellbeing of gay, lesbian, bisexual and transgender (GLBT) Australians. Melbourne: ARCSHS, La Trobe University.

Lowe, G. and Cristofis, L. (2017): The Australian Health System. In: The Journal for Nurse Practitioners, 13(8), p. 577.

McLean, A. (2011): A 'Gender Centre' for Melbourne? Assessing the Need for a Transgender Specific Service Provider. In: Gay and Lesbian Issues and Psychology Review, 7(1), pp. 33-42.

McNair, R.; Andrews, C.; Parkinson, S. and Dempsey, D. (2017): GALFA LGBTQ Homeless Research Project: Final Report. Melbourne: The University of Melbourne and Swinburne University of Technology.

Reeves, E. (2015): A Synthesis of the Literature on Trauma-Informed Care. In: Issues in Mental Health Nursing, 36(9), pp. 698-709.

Riggs, D. and Due, C. (2013): Gender Identity Australia: The healthcare experiences of people whose gender identity differs from that expected of their natally assigned sex. Adelaide: Flinders University.

Riggs, D.; Ansara, G. and Treharne, G. (2015): An Evidence-Based Model for Understanding the Mental Health Experiences of Transgender Australians. In: Australian Psychologist, 59(1), pp. 32-39.

Seelman, K.; Colon-Diaz, M.; LeCroix, R.; Xavier-Brier, M. and Kattari, L. (2017): Transgender Noninclusive Healthcare and Delaying Care Because of Fear: Connections to General Health and Mental Health Among Transgender Adults. In: Transgender Health, 2(1), pp. 17-28.

Smith, E.; Jones, T.; Ward, R.; Dixon, J.; Mitchell, A. and Hillier, L. (2014): From Blues to Rainbows: Mental health and wellbeing of gender diverse and transgender young people in Australia. Melbourne: The Australian Research Centre in Sex, Health and Society, La Trobe University.

Strauss, P.; Cook, A.; Winter, S.; Watson, V.; Wright Toussaint, D. and Lin, A. (2017): Trans Pathways: The Mental Health Experiences and Care Pathways of Trans Young People. Summary of Results. Perth: Telethon Kids Institute.

Stubbings, S.; Robb, K.; Waller, J.; Ramirez, A.; Austoker, J.; Macleod, U.; Hiom, S. and Wardle, J. (2009): Development of an awareness tool to assess public awareness of cancer. In: British Journal of Cancer, 101, pp. S13-S17.

Telfer, M.; Tollit, M. and Feldman, D. (2015): Transformation of health-care and legal systems for the transgender population: The need for change in Australia. In: Journal of Paediatrics and Child Health, 51(11), pp. 1051-1053.

Toone, K. (2015): Sistergirls and the Impact of Community and Family on Wellbeing. Adelaide: Flinders University.

Do Trans People Age Differently? Empirical Findings of International Studies on Trans Identities, Health and Age(ing) [1]

Max Nicolai Appenroth & Ralf Lottmann

It is evident that as life expectancy increases, the population of older adults will increase. Older Lesbian, Gay, Bisexual, and Trans people (LGBT) are becoming more visible. It is estimated that approximately five to ten percent of all seniors in the United States (US) identify as LGBT (Grant 2010). This means that within the next couple of decades, there will be two to seven million LGBT older adults in the US.

Little is known about older LGBT people, especially older people who do not identify with the gender they were assigned at birth and/or do not conform with stereotypical binary gender norms. This article focusses on the particular life circumstances, challenges, strengths and care needs of older trans people. While often discussed as a subset of the LGBT population overall, trans people have unique health needs and should be the focus of specific research within gerontology. Survey-based as well as anecdotal evidence indicates that the everyday reality of trans people differs from that of cisgender lesbian, gay and bisexual people in important ways, primarily due to the additional challenges imposed by hetero- and cis-normativity. The intention of the following article is to synthesize what is currently known about trans identities in aging and care.

---

[1] This article was first published in German in Appenroth, Max Nicolai and Castro Varela, María do Mar (eds.): Trans & Care: Trans Personen zwischen Selbstsorge, Fürsorge und Versorgung. Bielefeld: transcript. Minor changes/additions/updates were made to the original publication.

Trans Identities and Aging in Research

According to a survey from the Williams Institute at the University of California Los Angeles, approximately 1.4 million people (0.6% of adults) in the United States are trans (Flores et al. 2016:2). The number of gender questioning people is most likely higher than this. A recent study with data from Great Britain, New Zealand, Belgium, the Netherlands and the USA postulates that between 0.5 % and 1.2 % of the total population identify themselves as trans (Winter et al. 2016:392). The available studies show that the trans community seems to be dominated by young people. Rarely are persons over 54 years of age found in the results (James et al. 2016; FRA 2014). The experiences of this population group are usually "concealed" (Brown 2009). Established research on aging has rarely considered questions of gender diversity (Van Caenegem et al. 2015).

One reason for the underrepresentation of certain age groups might be the fact that most surveys have been conducted via online questionnaires[2]. It may be that socio-economic disadvantages that trans people face in their lives (see following section) influence their ability to access the internet at home. Some people may not feel comfortable taking part in specific surveys on shared computers or in shared spaces, where others could discover their gender identity. Besides this, age itself might play in important role in terms of the ability to use a computer and the internet. Invisibility of trans older adults may reflect a need for further efforts to reach out to this population and include them in research. It also may be that added to these disadvantages, poor general and mental health, and experiences of violence lead to an earlier death for many trans people, leading to their underrepresentation among older adults compared with LGB people and the non-LGBT population.

---

2   The usual age-related decline in participation in online surveys due to lack of Internet access and a lower affinity for technology (see File and Ryan 2014:3; Hanson 2001:14-15) could be less significant for the trans population than for the majority population, since the Internet is generally more important for trans people (among other things, due to the higher level of repression and lack of visibility, online social networks are more important). Socio-economic disadvantages could in turn be a reason why trans people have less frequent access to the Internet.

Challenges in the Life Course of Trans Identities

Socioeconomic Factors

Challenges and disadvantages throughout an individual's lifespan have great impact on the physical and mental health, general well-being, social life and socio-economic status. This section identified several areas in which trans people face higher disadvantages than cisgender LGB people and the general population[3]. These lifetime disadvantages speak to the importance of addressing trans people as their own target group in research about aging.

With regard to educational background, the analysis of the U.S. Transgender Survey (USTS; n=27,715), which reports on the lives of trans people in the United States, shows that trans people experience discrimination as early as school age and this discrimination often recurs throughout their lives. 17% of the respondents dropped out of school prematurely due to assaults and 6% were even expelled from school because of their gender identity. Those who continued to attend school found themselves in a violent environment. 77% report having been harassed, almost a quarter (24%) were subjected to physical violence and 13% experienced sexual violence (James et al. 2016:131).

Trans people are far more likely to belong to a low-income group or be living in poverty. In another study on U.S. trans identities (Injustice at Every Turn; n=6,450), 44% reported that they are "underemployed", i.e., despite good qualifications, they do not get adequate employment matching their qualifications (Grant et al. 2011:51). The USTS report states that 30% of the participants had lost their jobs, were not promoted or otherwise disadvantaged in the year prior to the study due to their gender identity. 15% were verbally or physically assaulted or sexually harassed at their workplace. 77% reported that they hid their identity or changed jobs because of the work climate. 27% reported that they had been disadvantaged in their search for a job (James et al. 2016:148) Similar numbers are found in the study "Being Trans in the European Union" (BTE study; n=6,579): According to this study, 37% of respondents stated that they had been discriminated against in their search for a job within the last 12 months. This is twice as often as lesbian, gay or bisexual participants experienced it. 27% were discriminated against in their workplace (FRA 2014:27). It is believed that trans people receive, on average,

---

3   We have used those studies that explicitly differentiate between sexual orientation and gender identity in their results and data evaluation.

lower incomes because of these experiences of discrimination (James et al. 2016:ff.; FRA 2014:121; Grant et al. 2011:2).

For example, the EU-wide BTE study, which is based on the methodology of the European Social Survey (ESS), reports that compared to LGB respondents in the study, trans people are more likely to receive income in the lowest quartile and less likely to receive income in the highest quartile (FRA 2014:20ff.). The results of the latest study (USTS) show that 29% of the participating trans people live in poverty. This is twice as high as in the US general population, where the overall poverty rate is 14 % (James et al. 2016:140). Even if only few older trans people participated in these studies, it is reasonable to assume that the situation for trans elders is similar, if not even worse.

Health Factors

In an online study (AH-Report; n=2,536) of the University of Washington conducted among older LGBT people in 2011 (AH Report; n=2,536), 174 participants (6.9% of all respondents) identified themselves as trans (Fredriksen-Goldsen et al. 2011:11). 47% of trans respondents stated that they suffered from depression, compared with 32% for LGB respondents, while 39% had anxiety, compared to 26% of LGB respondents (ibid.:26). In the USTS report, 40% of trans people reported having survived at least one suicide attempt, compared to 4.6% of the mainstream population. 82% reported having had suicidal thoughts at least once (James et al. 2016:112). In addition to these already alarming numbers, one third (33%) of the trans seniors surveyed in the AH-Report described poor general health and poor physical health. Compared to the cisgender LGB group, trans seniors are more likely to be physically disabled. The rate of trans people who are considered overweight in the AH-Report is 40%, which is significantly higher than for LGB people (26%), and indicates a higher risk of diabetes, coronary heart disease and osteoarthritis (Fredriksen-Goldsen et al. 2011:23-24). The above-mentioned aspects of education, work and mental health have a significant impact on well-being and on whether and how well a body can recover from discrimination-related stress. Studies on cis gay men show the extent to which social discrimination, socioeconomic status and minority stress influence mental well-being and the acquisition of mental illness (on gay men: Drewes and Kruspe 2016:82ff.; Drewes 2015). It is reasonable to assume that the impact of discrimination and minority stress on trans people is even greater, given the overall poorer profile of economic discrimination, general and mental health outcomes for this group.

Other negative factors for life expectancy and quality of life are that trans people are less likely to engage with preventive health examinations, and more at risk of Human Immunodeficiency Virus (HIV). 1.4% of the respondents in the USTS report stated that they were HIV positive, compared to 0.3 % of the U.S. population. Another 46% of respondents did not know their HIV status (James et al. 2016:4). Trans persons are more likely than cis persons to be drug users, more likely to be financially dependent on sex work and more likely to engage in unprotected sex (Grant et al. 2011:65; Auldridge et al. 2012:14-15; James et al. 2016:115).

At this point it should be noted that in the USA, having health insurance or receiving adequate medical care depends heavily on a person's financial resources. Trans people in the USA are particularly affected by insufficient healthcare provision due to lack of health insurance: 22% of the older trans people surveyed in the AH-Report stated that they could not afford to see a doctor in the 12 months prior to the study. Among LGB people of the same age this was 8% (Fredriksen-Goldsen et al. 2011:30). Trans seniors are also much less likely to undergo preventive examinations such as colonoscopy (LGB: 56.1% compared to trans: 42.2%) or osteoporosis screening (LGB: 32.9%, trans: 19.1%) (ibid.:73). 40% of trans people reported that they received inadequate care or were even denied medical assistance (11 % for LGBs) (ibid.:31).

Out of trans respondents to the USTS, 25% reported that they had been denied transition-related medical care and 33% of the respondents had to postpone a visit to a doctor despite illness or injury because they did not have the financial means during the 12 months prior to the study. Out of fear of discrimination, 23% of the participating trans persons did not go to a doctor and 33% reported negative experiences (e.g., refusal of medical care, discrimination) in their search for medical treatment (James et al. 2016:93). The EU-wide BTE study shows a very similar picture: 22% of the participants were discriminated against by medical personnel in the past 12 months because of their gender identity. For example, 26% of the respondents from Germany experienced discrimination in healthcare. These figures suggest that even a form of statutory health insurance such as the one found in Germany by no means guarantees adequate and barrier-free medical care for gender diverse people. In addition to these experiences of discrimination, about half of all participants in the USTS reported that their medical practitioner did not know about trans specific medical care (e.g., hormone administration or hormone-drug interactions) and the patient had to provide this information themself (ibid.:96). A similar picture can be found in Europe, where 30% of those surveyed reported that medical staff were willing to intervene appropriately but did not have any expertise in the care of trans people (see Whittle et al. 2008).

A related issue in trans medical care is trans people's dependence on health professionals not just for access to medical interventions such as hormone therapy, but also in the process of seeking legal recognition of their gender identities (Cook-Daniels 2016:294-295). In many countries, either a statement by a physician, or forced sterilization, is a prerequisite for legal recognition of a trans person's gender (i.e., changing the first name and/or gender maker in official documents). As a result, physicians can act as 'gatekeepers' preventing many trans people from achieving legal gender recognition. In the USTS, only 11% of the respondents reported having been able to change their first name and gender marker on official documents (James et al. 2016:82).[4] Many trans people who have not changed their legal name or gender are confronted with the danger of being 'forcibly outed' because their official documents do not match their gender presentation. Psychologists and psychiatrists may be similarly influential in determining whether a trans person is given access to hormone treatment or gender affirming surgeries. In many countries, access to these interventions requires diagnosis with a mental illness, contributing to further pathologization and stigmatization of trans experience (Cook-Daniels 2016:295).

Cook-Daniels (2016) discusses additional barriers that older trans people may face to accessing medical examinations or receiving assistance with personal care. Some trans people are able to exercise discretion about when, and to whom, to reveal their trans identity. However, particular medical and aged care procedures (i.e., receiving assistance with bathing), may require that the person providing the service sees the genitals of the person receiving the service. According to the above-mentioned NTDS report, only 21-23% of the male-to-female (MtF) and none of the female-to-male (FtM) respondents had undergone gender affirming bottom surgery, due to the large number of possible complications. Some trans people who have not undergone such surgeries face the risk of having their trans identity involuntarily revealed in the context of a medical examination or assisted personal care. Cook-Daniels observes that this reality may discourage trans seniors from seeking medical care (see under *Health Factors* above). Ignorance on the part of caregivers

---

4   It needs to be noted that not every trans person wants to legally change their given name and/or gender marker, nor does every trans person wish to undergo any other social, physical and/or legal changes.

about the treatment of trans people may be one reason why this group less often agrees to home care or placement in an inpatient facility, even if this is recommended to them (ibid.:294). Furthermore, it should be noted that even if a normative physical alignment has taken place, in the case of later nursing care, earlier transition-related surgical interventions require appropriate treatment. Visible scars, or required hormonal medication, may lead ignorant nursing staff to demand an explanation which can result in unwanted conversations about the individual's trans history.

(Family-)Networks

Further differences between trans people compared to cis LGB and non-LGBT people can also be found in social and family life. 18% of trans people interviewed said they were parents and 14% lived with a child in the same household, compared to 34% in the general population. Of those participants who lived their trans identity openly in front of their children, 21% said that the children did not talk to them because of that. In addition, 40% of all trans respondents did not receive positive support from their family (James et al. 2016:ff.). Even though trans seniors are more likely to have children than older cis LGB, the probability of feeling lonely is higher than in the cis LGB comparison group. In particular, rejection by the family and limited contact with one's own children, or even a break-off of contact, can lead to a life situation that is characterized by an above-average degree of isolation, especially in old age (Fredriksen-Goldsen et al. 2011). Nevertheless, a recent study by Erosheva et al. (2016) showed that trans seniors have more opportunities than cis LGB seniors to build a social network in diverse communities (ibid.:114). In the study of 1,913 older LGBT respondents, including 136 trans identified participants, trans seniors were found to have the largest network size (median=54.5). Other aspects of diversity that go beyond the category of gender identity, was also most prevalent in trans networks (under control of other variables, including network size) (ibid.:107ff.).

Discussion

The data presented reveal a variety of barriers to a good quality of life for trans seniors, which are rooted in the discrimination that is observed over the lifespan of gender diverse people. Older trans people who – like others – are confronted with challenges of old age, such as a reduction of their social network and increasing restriction of mobility, need a considerable number of coping strategies and social resources to deal with these challenges. Discrimination, a stressful environment at school and at work, financial worries, social exclusion, and a lack of medical care can lead to greater levels of psychological and physical stress. If we look at the studies by Fredriksen-Goldsen and others, the situation is only partially comparable to the lives of cis LGB seniors. Trans seniors are confronted with mental health problems and pathologizing, discriminatory experiences with medical professionals. Doctors and psychologists often misuse their power as decision-makers and gatekeepers during medical and legal procedures associated with transition (Fredriksen-Goldsen et al. 2011; FRA 2014; Elder 2016; Cook-Daniels 2016). Experiences in psychotherapeutic care that trans patients report in qualitative studies are often described as traumatic. A small improvement in trans people's experiences with psychotherapeutic support has been observed in recent years; however, there is still much more work to be done in this area (Elder 2016:182-183).

All of the lifelong challenges discussed above contribute to the disproportionate difficulties that trans seniors may face in accessing quality care in old age. The BTE study assumes that, due to the above-mentioned challenges and experiences in the healthcare system, this population group has the highest probability of recurring discrimination experiences among the subgroups under the umbrella of LGBT (FRA 2014).

Despite the almost incalculable experiences of discrimination, violence, rejection, and psychological problems, a recent study on trans and aging points out that trans seniors do not necessarily experience the phase of old age negatively, but rather assess their life situation as peaceful (Porter, Ronneberg and Witten 2013). This is made possible by personal identity development and the accomplishment of the developmental psychological task of ego integrity. Also, increased resilience due to overcoming life crises and the positive experience of self-activity in one's own social networks seem to work towards a positively experienced second half of life (Porter et al. 2016). Additional results of a qualitative study conducted in Germany[5] show how the diverse expressions of sexual and gender identities shape the lives of LGBT older adults who are in need of care. It became apparent that the experiences of everyday nursing care are directly influenced by biographical events and access to self-help structures for care receivers and reactions and

---

5   „GLEPA – Gleichgeschlechtliche Lebensweisen und Pflege im Alter", at the Alice Salomon University of Applied Sciences Berlin

attitudes of the carers. It was also observed that trans seniors in need of care make use of biographic experiences in order to act in self-determined ways in care settings (see Lottmann 2018).

From the LGBT community, concrete demands are sometimes formulated, which are used on the basis of the presented data for the further development of regular medical services. Advocacy for GLBT Elders (SAGE) and the National Center for Transgender Equality (Auldridge et al. 2012) have drawn up an action plan that shows how the needs of trans seniors can be better taken into account and their quality of life improved. In particular, they call for a culture of anti-discrimination through mission statements and the visibility of LGBT people in medical and nursing institutions. Additionally, they advocate for further education and training to improve the awareness of all medical personnel about the concerns and interests of trans people, especially regarding their rights to privacy, dignity and self-determination. In addition, as can be seen from the above-mentioned results on trans and HIV, trans senior citizens must be given special attention in HIV awareness campaigns, as they have been and are still exposed to a high risk of infection with HIV. Furthermore, some authors call for sanctions for misconduct or denial of services by medical providers (Auldridge et al. 2012:34ff.; Porter et al. 2016).

Due to the growing visibility of the aging trans community, both outpatient and inpatient geriatric care facilities will be confronted with this topic. Within the framework of the LGBT Senior Studies at the Alice Salomon University, knowledge of the living environments not only of older cis lesbians and cis gays, but also of trans people, was considered essential for a sufficient care quality (Linschoten et al. 2016). Understanding of LGBT issues by nursing staff is necessary to ensure that neither those in need of care nor their relatives have to hide. In this context, LGBT personnel in nursing homes are of great importance, as they are to be understood as a resource for these facilities. The "Pink Passkey" care quality label developed in the Netherlands is an instrument for implementing trans-sensitive care in both institutional and inpatient facilities, not only in metropolitan but also rural regions (see ibid.). In the development of diversity-sensitive care labels such as this, it is recommended that LGBT associations and organizations be involved (ibid.:239). Since spring 2018, the Schwulenberatung (Berlin Gay Council Center) has been offering the "Diversity Check" for the first time for care facilities. This is a quality seal created for the German care landscape, which was developed in cooperation with community organizations and is explicitly informed by trans life experiences and the needs of this community.

The limited empirical evidence on trans people in general means that there are still too few concrete recommendations for action for this vulnerable population group. Methodologically, the existing studies under the label LGBT do not differentiate between the respective population groups. Merely adding a 'T' to the chain of letters in order to appear inclusive or to postulate more comprehensive results is a common but insufficient practice. Instead of including that group, exactly the opposite happens: the invisibility of trans people is preserved and the everyday experiences of discrimination as well as the specific living conditions of this group of people are neglected. The experiences of LGB people in nursing care and, to a greater extent, the experiences of trans seniors with healthcare facilities make it clear that "the debate about how discrimination and experiences of discrimination are to be thought about is far from over. Even though many social scientists pretend that intersectional thinking is a standard procedure, we still encounter insufficient studies. For example, too many studies still speak of 'age(s)' without examining the intersections" (Castro Varela 2016:63). Scientific research has too often ignored the situation of LGB and trans people (Lautmann 2016:43; BMFSFJ 2016:68ff.). The perspective of trans seniors must finally find its way into nursing and aging research.

References

Auldridge, A.; Tamar-Mattis, A.; Kennedy, S.; Ames, E. and Tobin, H.J. (2012): Improving the Lives of Transgender Older Adults. Recommendations for Policy and Practice [online]. New York and Washington, DC: SAGE and National Center for Transgender Equality. Available at: https://transequality.org/sites/default/files/docs/resources/TransAgingPolicyReportFull.pdf (Accessed: 14 November 2021).

Bundesministerium für Familie, Senioren, Frauen und Jugend (BMFSFJ, 2016): Siebter Bericht zur Lage der älteren Generation in der Bundesrepublik Deutschland. Sorge und Mitverantwortung in der Kommune – Aufbau und Sicherung zukunftsfähiger Gemeinschaften. BT-Drs. 18/10210 [online]. Available at: https://dserver.bundestag.de/btd/18/102/1810210.pdf (Accessed: 14 November 2021).

Castro Varela, M. (2016): Altern Andere anders? Queere Reflexionen. In: Lottmann, R.; Lautmann, R. and Castro Varela, M. (Eds.): Homosexualität_en und Alter(n). Wiesbaden: Springer VS, pp. 51-67.

Cook-Daniels, L. (2016): Understanding Transgender Elders. In: Harley, D. and Teaster, P. (Eds.): Handbook of LGBT Elders – An Interdisciplinary Approach to Principles, Practices, and Policies. Cham, Heidelberg, New York, Dordrecht and London: Springer International Publishing, pp. 285-308.

Drewes, J. (2015): Gesundheit schwuler Männer. In: Kolip, P. and Hurrelmann, K. (Eds.): Handbuch Geschlecht und Gesundheit: Männer und Frauen im Vergleich. Bern: Huber, pp. 409-419.

Drewes, J. and Kruspe, M. (2016): Schwule Männer und HIV/AIDS 2013. Schutzverhalten und Risikomanagement in den Zeiten der Behandelbarkeit von HIV. Abschlussbericht zu einer Befragung im Auftrag der Bundeszentrale für gesundheitliche Aufklärung [online]. Köln: Deutsche AIDS-Hilfe. Available at: https://www.aidshilfe.de/shop/pdf/7850 (Accessed 14 November 2021).

Elder, A.B. (2016): Experiences of Older Transgender and Gender Nonconforming Adults in Psychotherapy: A Qualitative Study. In: Psychology of Sexual Orientation and Gender Diversity, 3(2), pp. 180-186.

Erosheva, E.; Kim, H.J.; Emlet, C. and Fredriksen-Goldsen, K. (2016): Social Networks of Lesbian, Gay, Bisexual, and Transgender Older Adults. In: Research on Aging, 38(1), pp. 98-123.

European Agency of Fundamental Rights (FRA, 2013): EU LGBT Survey. European Union Lesbian, Gay, Bisexual and Transgender Survey. Results at a Glance [online]. Available at: https://fra.europa.eu/sites/default/files/eu-lgbt-survey-results-at-a-glance_en.pdf (Accessed: 14 November 2021).

European Agency of Fundamental Rights (FRA, 2014): Being Trans in the European Union. Comparative analysis of EU LGBT survey data [online]. Available at: https://fra.europa.eu/sites/default/files/eu-lgbt-survey-results-at-a-glance_en.pdf (Accessed: 14 November 2021).

File, T. and Ryan, C. (2014): Computer and Internet Use in the United States: 2013. American Community Survey Reports [online]. Washington DC: U.S. Census Bureau. Available at: https://www.census.gov/history/pdf/acs-internet2013.pdf (Accessed: 14 November 2021).

Flores, A.; Herman, J.; Gates, G. and Brown, T. (2016): How Many Adults Identify as Transgender in the United States [online]. Los Angeles, CA: The Williams Institute. Available at: https://williamsinstitute.law.ucla.edu/wp-content/uploads/Trans-Adults-US-Aug-2016.pdf (Accessed: 14 November 2021).

Fredriksen-Goldsen, K.; Kim, H.J.; Emlet, C.; Muraco, A.; Erosheva, E.; Hoy-Ellis, C.; Goldsen, J. and Petry, H. (2011): The Aging and Health Report. Disparities and Resilience among Lesbian, Gay, Bisexual, and Transgender Older Adults [online]. Seattle: Institute for Multigenerational Health. Available at: https://www.familleslgbt.org/1463149763/Fredriksen-Goldsen%202011.pdf (Accessed: 14 November 2021).

Grant, J.; Mottet, L.; Tanis, J.; Harrison, J.; Herman, J. and Keisling, M. (2011): Injustice at Every Turn. A Report of the National Transgender Discrimination Survey [online]. Washington, DC: National Center for Transgender Equality and National Gay and Lesbian Task Force. Available at: https://transequality.org/sites/default/files/docs/resources/NTDS_Report.pdf (Accessed: 14 November 2021).

Grant, J. (2010): Outing Age2010 – Public Policiy Issues Affecting Lesbian, Gay, Bisexual, and Transgender Elders [online]. Available at: https://www.lgbtagingcenter.org/resources/pdfs/OutingAge2010.pdf (Accessed: 31 January 2022).

Hanson, V. (2001): Web Access for Elderly Citizens. In: Proceedings of the 2001 EC/NFS workshop on Universal accessibility of ubiquitous computing: providing for the elderly. New York: Association for Computing Machinery, pp. 14-18.

James, S.; Herman, J.; Rankin, S.; Keisling, M.; Mottet, L. and Anafi, M. (2016): The Report of the 2015 U.S. Transgender Survey [online]. Washington, DC: National Center for Transgender Equality. Available at: https://transequality.org/sites/default/files/docs/usts/USTS-Full-Report-Dec17.pdf (Accessed: 14 November 2021).

Lautmann, R. (2016): Die soziokulturelle Lebensqualität von Lesben und Schwulen im Alter. In: Lottmann, R.; Lautmann, R. and Castro Varela, M. (Eds.): Homosexualität_en und Alter(n). Wiesbaden: Springer VS, pp. 15-50.

Linschoten, M.; Lottmann, R. and Lauscher, F. (2016): „The Pink Passkey®" – ein Zertifikat für die Verbesserung der Akzeptanz von LSBT*I-Pflegebedürftigen in Pflegeeinrichtungen. In: Lottmann, R.; Lautmann, R. and Castro Varela, M. (Eds.): Homosexualität_en und Alter(n). Wiesbaden: Springer VS, pp. 233-241.

Lottmann, R. (2018): LSBT*I-Senior*innen in der Pflege: Zu Relevanz und Besonderheiten sozialer Netzwerke und der Arbeit mit Angehörigen. In: Pflege & Gesellschaft, 23(3), pp. 228-244.

Porter, K.; Ronneberg, C. and Witten, T. (2013): Religious Affiliation and Successful Aging among Transgender Older Adults: Findings from the Trans MetLife Survey. In: Journal of Religion, Spirituality & Aging, 25(2), pp. 112-138.

Porter, K.; Brennan-Ing, M.; Chang, S.; Dickey, L.; Singh, A.; Bower, K. and Witten, T. (2016): Providing Competent and Affirming Services for Transgender and Gender Nonconforming Older Adults. In: Clinical Gerontologist, 39(5), pp. 366-388.

Van Caenegem, E.; Wierckx, K.; Elaut, E.; Buysse, A.; Dewaele, A.; Van Nieuwerburgh, F.; De Cuypere, G. and T'Sjoen, G. (2015): Prevalence of Gender Nonconformity in Flanders, Belgium. In: Archives of Sexual Behavior, 44(5), pp. 1281-1287.

Whittle, S.; Turner, L.; Combs, R. und Rhodes, S. (2008): Transgender EuroStudy: Legal Survey and Focus on the Transgender Experience of Health Care [online]. Brussels and Berlin: ILGA Europe and Transgender Europe. Available at: https://www.researchgate.net/publication/242527 943_Transgender_EuroStudy_Legal_Survey_and_Focus_on_the_Transg ender_Experience_of_Health_Care_Written_by (Accessed: 14 November 2021).

Winter, S.; Diamond, M.; Green, J.; Karasic, D.; Reed, T.; Whittle, S. and Wylie, K. (2016): Transgender People: Health at the Margins of Society. In: The Lancet, 388(10042), pp. 390-400.

About the authors (in order of appearance in the book)

Max Appenroth (they/he) is a Germany-based trans activist, diversity consultant, and in the final year of their PhD at the Institute of Public Health at the Charité Universitätsmedizin Berlin, Germany. Max is an internationally recognized expert in HIV prevention and care for trans and gender diverse communities and has worked with WHO, UNAIDS, the Robert Koch Institute, GATE, AVAC, among other organizations and institutions. With their own company 'diversity sparq' Max offers workshops and trainings to companies, institutions, and (health)care facilities to learn (more) about sexual and gender diversity, and how to make workplaces and services more inclusive and accessible. More information: www.max-appenroth.com

María do Mar Castro Varela (she/her) is a professor of Pedagogy and Social Work at the Alice Salomon University of Applied Science in Berlin with focus on Gender and Queer Studies. She holds a double degree in Psychology and Pedagogy and a PhD in Political Science. In 2021/22 she was the Sir Peter Ustinov Visiting Professor at the Institute of Contemporary History at the University of Vienna. Her work focuses on queer studies, postcolonial theory, critical migration and educational studies, trauma, and conspiracy narratives. Amongst others, she was Senior Fellow at the Institute for the Science of Man (IWM) in Vienna in 2015/16. She is the founder of bildungsLab* (bildungslab.net) and chair of the Berlin Institute for Contrapuntal Social Analysis.

Anahí Farji Neer (she/her) (Ph.D.) is a Postdoctoral Fellow at Gino Germani Research Institute of the Buenos Aires University, Argentina. Anahí Farji Neer received her Ph.D. in Social Sciences, her Master's Degree in Social Science Research and her B.A. in Sociology from the University of Buenos Aires, Argentina. Her doctoral dissertation titled "Debating the meanings of the trans bodies: medical, judicial, activist, and parliamentary discourses in Argentina (1966-2015)", focused on discourses related to the construction of trans bodies in Argentina between 1966 and 2015. There, she analyzed and compared discursive productions in the medical, legal, activist and parliamentary fields. Her current research consists in studying the discourses produced in the medical field as they relate to the bodily desires and the autonomous decisions of trans people.

Alex Rodrigo Castillo Hernández (he/him) is a trans man born in Guatemala City, a husband, father, and grandfather. He is a professional business administrator and human rights defender of the LGTBI population. Alex found the 1st collective of Trans Men in Central America called 'Trans-Formation' in 2013. He is the president of the Central American Network of Trans Men since 2014 and a former member of the Grant Making Panel of the International Trans Fund.

Yusimil Carrazana Hernandez (she/her) is a cis woman, family doctor and surgeon, of Cuban nationality and with an affiliation at the University of San Carlos of Guatemala. She has more than 30 years of experience in her field and works for the trans population under the Standards of Care of the WPATH 7th version. Email: yusicarrazana@gmail.com

Yana Kirey-Sitnikova (she/her) is a trans activist, independent consultant, and researcher from Russia. In 2021, she graduated from the University of Gothenburg, Sweden with a Master's degree in Public Health.

Carter Honoree (he/him) is currently part of the Board of Directors of Transgender Europe (TGEU) and was the Regional Coordinator for Africa in the TvT-TGEU (Transrespect versus Transphobia) project. He is a founder and was the Executive Director of Rwanda's Gender Pride, a trans feminist and non-binary organization in Rwanda. This organization specifically focused on the access to HIV services and prevention for trans MSM in Rwanda. Carter also served as a member of the Grant Making Panel (GMP) of the International Trans Fund (ITF) and was part of the Peer Grant Committee (PGC) in the UHAI East African Sexual Human Rights Initiative. Carter is currently supporting the project lead and coordination of the BIPOC and racial justice strand within Ulex.

Michael Aondo-verr Kombol (he/him) is a trans activist, university professor at the Benue State University and the Executive Director of Rural Renewal and Community Health Development Initiative (RURCHEDI), Makurdi Nigeria. Apart from partnerships with Heartland Alliance International, Nigeria (HAI-N) and the AIDS Prevention Initiative in Nigeria (APIN) on the CDC funded ICares project to provide HIV treatment to vulnerable populations, RURCHEDI, he researches issues around the treatment of sexually transmitted infections (STIs) among hard-to-reach populations (incl. trans people).

Elma de Vries (she/they) is a family physician working in primary care in Cape Town, South Africa, a lecturer in Family Medicine at the University of Cape Town, and a member of the Groote Schuur Transgender clinic team. Elma is currently doing a PhD with the topic, "How can the professional identity formation of a gender-affirming practitioner inform medical curriculum change?".

Chris/tine McLachlan (she/he/they) is a clinical psychologist in the public and private sector and a PhD candidate at the University of South Africa. Chris has published academic articles and presented papers locally and internationally and was the runner-up of the WPATH student award in 2018. Chris serves on various boards of NPO's focusing on trans and gender diversity and trains in the field of sexuality and gender diversity.

Trans* Ratgeber Kollektiv is an initiative of trans people, friends and supporters of trans people in closed settings, like prisons or psychiatric institutions. With their work and publications, they aim to support, to build a network, and to spread information among incarcerated trans and gender diverse people. More information: www.transundhaft.blogsport.de/

Aedan Wolton (he/they) is a social worker and trans health advocate with over a decade of experience in the HIV sector. He worked to design and establish the TransPlus service at 56 Dean Street and is a regular contributor to community-led research focused on exploring and improving trans health and wellbeing.

Matthew Hibbert (he/him) graduated from his PhD at Liverpool John Moores University in 2020 studying sexualised drug use among LGBT people. He previously worked for Public Health England in the HIV/STI department, working on HIV epidemiology and specializing in LGB and trans inclusion.

Sasha Strong (they/them) is a psychotherapist in private practice in Portland, Oregon, USA, and a doctoral candidate at the California Institute of Integral Studies. Their research focuses on bipolar disorder, mindfulness, Buddhism, psychotherapy, and trans, non-binary, and gender diverse people.

Sagan Wallace (they/them) is the evening supervisor at Oregon State University, USA, and a graduate student of information science at San José State University, USA. Their research interests include citizen science, digital privacy, and social justice initiatives.

Caleb Feldman (he/him, they/them) is adjunct faculty at Clackamas Community College and Clark College, where he teaches geography. His research interests include climate justice and educational equity.

Ruby J. Welch (she/her, they/them) is a part-time musician and full-time teacher's assistant in Portland Oregon. Their stage persona, Ruby Q, enjoys showtunes and picture books, and shares them on social media as @rubyqpdx.

Jeremy A. Gottlieb (they/them) is an MD-PhD Student in Medical Anthropology at the University of California, San Francisco and the University of California, Berkeley. They graduated *cum laude* in 2018 from Duke University with a B.A. with honors in Cultural Anthropology. Jeremy identifies as gender non-conforming.

Omer Elad (they/them) has been an activist and a leader in the trans and queer communities for nearly two decades. Once an artist turned a social worker, they have primarily worked in the intersection of mental health and homelessness in Boston, Massachusetts and Portland, Oregon in the United States. Utilizing intersectionality as a main framework, they continue to navigate their own various identities as an anti-occupation Israeli, a white immigrant of middle-class background, disabled, non-binary and very queer person, and how those all fit (or not) within their capacity as a change maker, mental health provider and supervisor.

Brenda Rodriguez Alegre (she/her) (Ph.D.) is a transpinay based in Hong Kong. She is a lecturer in Gender Studies at The University of Hong Kong. She is also on the Board of ILGA Asia, STRAP and Planet Ally. Her teaching and research focus is on trans issues, intersectionality, migration, health and histories. She is also a choir soprano.

Lucille Kerr (she/her) is a Ph.D. candidate at the Australian Research Centre in Sex, Health and Society, La Trobe University, Melbourne. She is also a research fellow at a Department of Nursing Research, specialist cancer nurse and completed her Bachelor of Nursing with Honours at the University of Tasmania.

Christopher M. Fisher (he/him) (B.A., A.A., M.A., Ph.D.) is an Associate Professor and takes a leading role in research on young peoples' sexual health and wellbeing. A major focus of the work is on adolescent sexual health knowledge, behaviors and educational experiences (both formal and informal). He leads the National Survey of Secondary Students and Sexual Health in Australia. Previous work has looked at the role of youth development professionals in Non-Governmental Organizations (e.g., youth groups) in providing sexual health information as well as adolescent perspectives on promoting sexual health. He has also conducted population-based research in LGBTIQ health and HIV prevention and care.

Tiffany Jones (she/her) (B.CA., Bed-Hons1, Ph.D.) is an Associate Professor and sociologist who researches LGBTIQ+ issues in education, education policy, health and social policy. Her projects have been supported by the ARC (DECRA, Linkage), UNESCO, beyondblue, governments and many other bodies. Her new releases include 'Improving Services for Transgender and Gender Variant Youth', 'A Student-centred Sociology of Education' and 'Bent Street vol.4.2'.

Ralf Lottman (he/him) has studied Sociology in Berlin and Gerontology in Amsterdam. He has worked for care providers and the German Parliament before moving on to research projects at the Alice Salmon University of Applied Sciences in Berlin (D) and the University of Surrey (UK). He is now Professor of Health Policy at Magdeburg-Stendal University of Applied Sciences.

Social Sciences

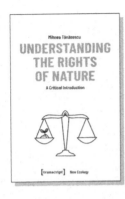

Mihnea Tanasescu
Understanding the Rights of Nature
A Critical Introduction

February 2022, 168 p., pb.
40,00 € (DE), 978-3-8376-5431-8
E-Book: available as free open access publication
PDF: ISBN 978-3-8394-5431-2

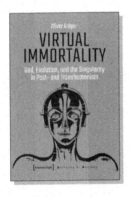

Oliver Krüger
**Virtual Immortality –
God, Evolution, and the Singularity
in Post- and Transhumanism**

2021, 356 p., pb., ill.
35,00 (DE), 978-3-8376-5059-4
E-Book:
PDF: 34,99 (DE), ISBN 978-3-8394-5059-8

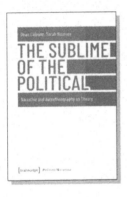

Dean Caivano, Sarah Naumes
The Sublime of the Political
Narrative and Autoethnography as Theory

2021, 162 p., hardcover
100,00 (DE), 978-3-8376-4772-3
E-Book:
PDF: 99,99 (DE), ISBN 978-3-8394-4772-7

**All print, e-book and open access versions of the titles in our list
are available in our online shop www.transcript-publishing.com**

Social Sciences

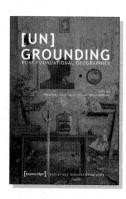

Friederike Landau, Lucas Pohl, Nikolai Roskamm (eds.)
[Un]Grounding
Post-Foundational Geographies

2021, 348 p., pb., col. ill.
50,00 (DE), 978-3-8376-5073-0
E-Book:
PDF: 49,99 (DE), ISBN 978-3-8394-5073-4

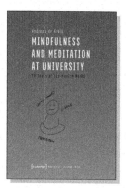

Andreas de Bruin
Mindfulness and Meditation at University
10 Years of the Munich Model

2021, 216 p., pb.
25,00 (DE), 978-3-8376-5696-1
E-Book: available as free open access publication
PDF: ISBN 978-3-8394-5696-5

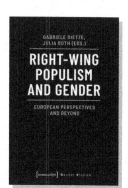

Gabriele Dietze, Julia Roth (eds.)
Right-Wing Populism and Gender
European Perspectives and Beyond

2020, 286 p., pb., ill.
35,00 (DE), 978-3-8376-4980-2
E-Book:
PDF: 34,99 (DE), ISBN 978-3-8394-4980-6

**All print, e-book and open access versions of the titles in our list
are available in our online shop www.transcript-publishing.com**